Central Service
Technical Manual Workbook

Eighth Edition

The Central Service Technical Manual Workbook is designed to provide a better understanding of the information presented in the Central Service Technical Manual, Eighth Edition. This workbook includes chapter practice exercises, chapter quizzes, and progress tests.

A variety of question formats are utilized in this workbook (true/false, short answer, matching, etc) which offer the opportunity to practice knowledge of key Central Service topics and concepts most important to a successful Central Service technician.

Please keep in mind that the CRCST certification exam is comprised of only multiple choice questions. The exact questions in this workbook will not appear on the CRCST certification exam.

The CRCST Exam Content Outline is another study tool which details each of the seven domains that comprise the CRCST exam, as well as the various topics which are covered under each section. The CRCST Exam Content Outline can be found in the Certification section of the IAHCSMM website.

©2016
By the International Association of Healthcare
Central Service Materiel Management
55 West Wacker Drive, Suite 501
Chicago, IL 60601

The International Association of Healthcare Central Service Materiel Management is a non-profit corporation.

Printed in the United States of America

ISBN 978-1-4951-8905-0

TABLE OF CONTENTS

Chapter 1
Introduction to Central Service

Learning Objectives

As a result of successfully completing this chapter, users will be able to:

1. Explain the importance of the Central Service department, with an emphasis on the service provided and the role of Central Service quality patient care

2. Review the work flow process in an effectively organized Central Service department

3. Identify basic knowledge and skills required for effective Central Service technicians

4. Define job responsibilities of Central Service technicians

5. Discuss the role of education and training in the field of Central Service

Reading Assignment

Read Chapter 1 in the *Central Service Technical Manual, Eighth Edition.*

Chapter 1: Practice Exercises

Indicate whether each of the following statements is true or false.

1. Since Central Service technicians do not handle money, ethics considerations do not apply to them.
   a. True
   b. False *(circled)*

2. Central Service technicians practice resource management when they control costs and reduce waste.
   a. True *(circled)*
   b. False

3. Central Service technicians must be able to identify approximately 100 surgical instruments in order to be proficient in their job.
   a. True
   b. False *(circled)*

4. Central Service technicians must be able to adapt to change.
   a. True *(circled)*
   b. False

5. Because all Central Service departments are structured alike, healthcare facilities use one standard job description for all Central Service technicians.
   a. True
   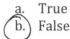 b. False

6. Career growth and progression is virtually nonexistent for Central Service technicians.
   a. True
    b. False

7. Departments that perform Central Service functions may go by other names at different facilities; for example, Sterile Processing and Distribution or Surgical Supply.
    a. True
   b. False

8. Central Service workflow can be divided into the handling of three categories of items: soiled items, clean items and sterile items.
   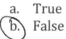 a. True
   b. False

9. The use of good verbal communication skills is the most important and most used skill for Central Service technicians to provide or obtain information.
   a. True
   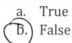 b. False

10. Since modern Central Service departments are virtually risk free, Central Service technicians need not be concerned with safety practices.
   a. True
    b. False

Chapter 1: Quiz

Turn to page 95 to complete the end of chapter review quiz.

Chapter 2
Medical Terminology for Central Service Technicians

 Learning Objectives

As a result of successfully completing this chapter, users will be able to:

1. Explain the importance of medical terminology for Central Service technicians

2. Identify the various elements used in medical terminology including prefixes, roots and suffixes

3. Discuss how medical terminology can refer to the human anatomy, disease processes, surgical instruments and surgical procedures

4. Understand medical terminology used to refer to surgical procedures in surgery schedules

5. Understand the importance of medical terminology for service quality in the Operating Room

 Reading Assignment

Read Chapter 2 in the *Central Service Technical Manual, Eighth Edition.*

 Chapter 2: Practice Exercises

Part One: Working with Prefixes

Practice using prefixes learned in this chapter by filling in the blanks.

1. The prefix *hyper-* means __ABOVE__ while the prefix *hypo-* means __UNDER__.

2. The prefix *para-* means __BESIDE__ while the prefix *peri-* means __AROUND__.

3. The prefix *inter-* means __BETWEEN__ while the prefix *intra-* means __INSIDE__.

4. The prefix *anti-* means __AGINST__ while the prefix *ante-* means __BEFORE__.

3

5. Match the prefixes with their meanings.

_D_ *endo-*   a. half
_A_ *hemi-*   b. above
_F_ *neo-*   c. without
_C_ *a-*   d. within
_E_ *post-*   e. after
_B_ *supra-*   f. new

Part Two: Working with Suffixes

Practice using suffixes learned in this chapter by filling in the blanks.

1. The suffix *-ostomy* means ___create an opening___ while the suffix *-otomy* means ___cut into___.

2. The suffix *-ectomy* means ___removal___ while the suffix *-oscopy* means ___viewing___.

3. The suffix *-cide* means ___to kill___ while the suffix *-cise* means ___cut___.

4. Name the three suffixes that mean *pertaining to*:_____,

_____ and _____.

Part Three: Working with Roots

Match the roots with their meanings by placing the letter of the meaning with the correct root.

___ *cardio*   a. skull

___ *chole*   b. skin

___ *cranio*   c. uterus/womb

___ *cysto*   d. liver

___ *derma*   e. fat

___ *gastro*   f. bile

___ *gyne*   g. stomach

___ *hepat*   h. nose

___ *herni*   i. stone

___ *hyster*   j. joint

___ *lipo*   k. rupture

___ *litho*   l. bladder

___ *rhino*   m. woman

___ *arthro*   n. heart

Part Four: Working with Abbreviations

Define the following abbreviations.

1. ORIF _____

2. BSO _____

3. BKA _____

4. CABG _____

5. THA _____

6. TAH _____

7. CR _____

Part Five: Working with Definitions

Define the purpose of each of the following three procedures.

1. Cholecystectomy   _____

2. Hysterectomy   _____ _____

3. Prostatectomy   _____

Part Six: Working with Terminology

Practice using terminology learned in this chapter by filling in the blanks.

1. A surgical procedure to examine the thoracic cavity is called a

_____ while the procedure to remove a lung is called a

_____.

2. The surgical procedure to visually examine a joint is called an

_____while the procedure to visually examine organs

of the abdomen is called a _____.

3. A colostomy is a procedure to _____ while a colectomy is a

procedure to _____.

4. A hysteroscopy is a _____ while a hysterectomy is a

procedure to _____.

 Chapter 2: Quiz
Turn to page 97 to complete the end of chapter review quiz.

Chapter 3
Anatomy for Central Service Technicians

 Learning Objectives

As a result of successfully completing this chapter, users will be able to:

1. Review the structure, function, activities and role of cells, tissues and organs in the body

2. Identify and describe the structure and roles of each major body system and identify common surgical procedures that involve each system:
    *   Skeletal
    *   Muscular
    *   Nervous
    *   Endocrine
    *   Reproductive
    *   Urinary and excretory
    *   Respiratory
    *   Digestive
    *   Circulatory

3. Explain how knowledge of anatomy can help with surgical instrument identification

 Reading Assignment

Read Chapter 3 in the *Central Service Technical Manual, Eighth Edition.*

 Chapter 3: Practice Exercises

Part One: Working with Names.

On the following two pages, read the description then fill in the surgical procedure being described and the body system on which the procedure is performed.

Description	Procedure	Body System
Example: *Making an opening into the skull to access the brain.*	*Craniotomy*	*Skeletal*
1. Making an opening into the thoracic cavity to give surgeons access to the lungs and heart.		
2. Removing a salivary gland because of a tumor formation.		
3. Removing plaque from the carotid artery that causes lack of brain oxygen.		
4. Removing a vein from the lower limb to bypass a blocked coronary artery of the heart.		
5. Removal of a kidney.		
6. Making an incision into the tympanic membrane (ear drum) to permit fluid to drain and placing small tubes in the membrane to permit continuous drainage.		
7. A repair to the muscles and ligaments of the shoulder joint.		
8. Removing disc tissue pressing on the lower spine area, inserting a piece of bone between the vertebras and fusing the area with plates and screws.		
9. Removing lymph tissue in the pharynx (throat).		
10. Removing the gall bladder.		
11. Straightening or removing cartilage and/or bone in the nose when the nasal septum is deformed, injured or fractured.		
12. Removing both fallopian tubes and ovaries.		
13. Removing tissue or displaced bone in the wrist area to release pressure on the median nerve.		

14. Moving an undescended testicle.		
15. Reconstructing the ear drum so sound waves can be sent to the middle and inner ear.		

Part Two: Matching

Match words and definitions using the list below (there will be more word selections than needed).

a. Cerebellum
b. Ovaries
c Liver
d. Brain stem
e. Pituitary gland
f. Prostate gland
g. Veins
h. Blood
i. Heart
j. Joint
k. Brain
l. Uterus
m. Skin

n. Tendon
o. Cell
p. Ureters
q. Calcification
r. Mouth
s. Arteries
t. Cerebrum
u. Cytoplasm
v. Alimentary canal
w. Ossification
x. Kidney
y. Esophagus
z. Thyroid gland

___ 1. This organ pumps blood throughout the body.

___ 2. The process by which cartilage is replaced by bone.

___ 3. Any place where two bones meet.

___ 4. The main control unit of the central nervous system.

___ 5. Considered the master gland because it helps control the activities of all other endocrine glands.

___ 6. This organ filters blood to remove amino acids and neutralize some harmful toxins.

___ 7. Produces a fluid element in semen that stimulates motility of sperm.

___ 8. The largest part of the brain; controls mental activities and movement.

___ 9. These carry blood away from the heart.

___ 10. A somewhat flexible tube that helps move food into the stomach.

___ 11. A type of connective tissue fluid that moves throughout the circulatory system.

___ 12. The pathway that food takes through the digestive system.

___ 13. Female reproductive organs.

___ 14. A cord of fibrous tissue that connects a muscle to a bone.

___ 15. The largest organ of the body.

___ 16. The basic unit of life.

___ 17. Tube-like structures that connect the kidneys to the urinary bladder.

___ 18. This is where the digestive process begins.

___ 19. Clear jelly-like substance that surrounds the nucleus of a cell.

___ 20. This part of the nervous system controls many automatic body functions like the heartbeat and breathing.

Chapter 3: Quiz

Turn to page 101 to complete the end of chapter review quiz.

Chapter 4
Microbiology for Central Service Technicians

Learning Objectives

As a result of successfully completing this chapter, users will be able to:

1. Define the term "microbiology" and explain why it is important for Central Service professionals to have a basic understanding of its science

2. Restate basic facts about microorganisms

3. Identify common ways to identify and classify microorganisms by:
   - Shape
   - Color change
   - Need for oxygen

4. Explain environmental conditions necessary for bacterial growth and survival

5. Provide basic information about non-bacterial organisms:
   - Viruses
   - Protozoa
   - Fungi
   - Prions

6. Review basic procedures to control and eliminate microorganisms

Reading Assignment

Read Chapter 4 in the *Central Service Technical Manual, Eighth Edition.*

Chapter 4: Practice Exercises

On the following page, recall key facts about microbiology by completing each sentence.

1.   The controlling unit of a cell that governs activity and heredity is called the

      _____.

2.   Pseudomonas is sometimes called the _____ because it is frequently found in water.

3.   _____ are often pathogenic to humans because they grow best at body temperature.

4.   Herpes simplex is a _____ disease.

5.   Bacteria that require free oxygen to grow are called _____ bacteria.

6.   Bacteria are divided into three main shape classifications: _____ (round),

      _____ (rods) and _____ (spirals).

7.   Microorganisms that are capable of forming a thick wall around them to survive in
      adverse conditions are called

      _____.

8.   The two most common processes designed to classify bacteria by color change are the

      _____ and the _____.

9.   Tetanus and botulism do not require free oxygen to grow, so they are classified as

      _____ bacteria.

10.   Using gram-stain classifications, *Staphylococcus*, *Enterococcus* and *Streptococcus* are

      examples of gram- _____ bacteria.

11.   The bacterial reproductive process that takes place when a mother cell divides into
      two daughter cells is called

      _____.

12.   Creutzfeldt-Jakob disease is caused by _____ which are believed to be

      _____.

13.   _____ is defined as the state of being soiled or infected by
      contact with infectious organisms or other material.

14.   Most bacteria are approximately _____ microns in size.

15.   Sunlight is lethal to the _____ stage of pathogens.

Chapter 4: Quiz
Turn to page 105 to complete the end of chapter review quiz.

PROGRESS TEST ONE

Turn to page 179 to complete **Progress Test One** before continuing on to Chapter 5.

Chapter 5
Regulations and Standards

Learning Objectives

As a result of successfully completing this chapter, users will be able to:

1. Explain the difference between regulations, voluntary standards and regulatory standards

2. Provide basic information about the U.S. Food and Drug Administration and other government and regulatory agencies

3. Explain the roles and responsibilities of the regulatory agencies that impact how the Central Service Department functions

4. Discuss how organizations and associations that develop regulations and standards affect Central Service

Reading Assignment

Read Chapter 5 in the *Central Service Technical Manual, Eighth Edition.*

Chapter 5: Practice Exercises

On the following page, match the statement with the correct letter for the agency or organization listed below (letters may be used more than once).

Then indicate whether the agency is voluntary (V) or regulatory (R) by circling the correct letter beneath each statement.

a. Centers for Disease Control
b. International Standards Organization
c. U.S. Food and Drug Administration
d Association for Professionals in Infection Control and Epidemiology
e. Department of Transportation
f. World Health Organization
g. Occupational Safety and Health Administration
h. Society of Gastroenterology Nurses and Associates
i. Association for the Advancement of Medical Instrumentation
j. Environmental Protection Agency
k. The Joint Commission
l. Association of periOperative Registered Nurses
m. United States Pharmacopeia–National Formulary
n. American National Standards Institute
o. National Fire Protection Association

___ 1. This organization specializes in endoscopy issues and has established standards for the effective processing of flexible endoscopes.
V   R

___ 2. Furthers international cooperation in improving health conditions.
V   R

___ 3. Develops nationally recognized guidelines for the perioperative setting.
V   R

___ 4. Protects workers from occupationally-caused illnesses and injuries.
V   R

___ 5. Proposed standards are submitted from members such as Association for the Advancement of Medical Instrumentation.
V   R

___ 6. Provides standards and evaluations for healthcare facilities. These evaluations are in the form of onsite surveys at least every three years.
V   R

___ 7. Creates and revises standards for processing water for irrigation.
V   R

___   8.   Creates and enforces laws relating to cleaner water, air and land.
            V   R

___   9.   A voluntary international organization dedicated to the prevention
            and control of infections and related outcomes.
            V   R

___   10.   Enforces laws relating to the transportation of medical waste.
            V   R

___   11.   Is considered one of the major resources for healthcare guidelines.
            V   R

___   12.   International standards to reduce the burden of fire and other
            hazards.
            V   R

___   13.   Promotes health by preventing and controlling disease.
            V   R

___   14.   Responsible for pre- and post-market medical device requirements,
            MedWatch, medical device classification and medical device recall.
            V   R

___   15.   Enhances the global competitiveness and quality of life by
            promoting standards and ensuring their integrity.
            V   R

__&__ 16.   Agencies responsible for regulating ethylene oxide.
            V   R

___   17.   Agency responsible for the MedWatch program.
            V   R

Chapter 5: Quiz
Turn to page 107 to complete the end of chapter review quiz.

Chapter 6
Infection Prevention

Learning Objectives

As a result of successfully completing this chapter, users will be able to:

1. Explain the role of Central Service in the prevention of healthcare-associated surgical infections

2. Explain the principles, practice and importance of personal hygiene and attire including personal protective equipment

3. Identify the hazards of bloodborne pathogens and how the Occupational Safety and Health Administration's requirements impact personal safety

4. Explain the rationale for the separation of clean and dirty, and the environmental requirements for maintaining that separation

5. Discuss the chain of infection and the technician's role in breaking that chain

Reading Assignment

Read Chapter 6 in the *Central Service Technical Manual, Eighth Edition.*

Chapter 6: Practice Exercises

Part One: Use the diagram below to list the proper attire required to work in each area.

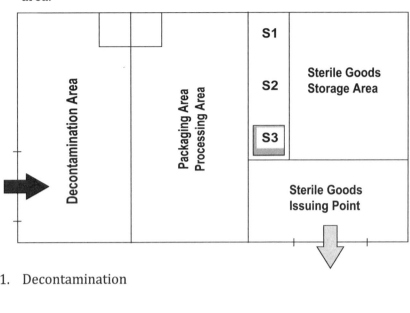

1. Decontamination

    _____

    _____

    _____

2. Packaging area/processing area

    _____

    _____

    _____

3. Sterile goods storage area

    _____

    _____

    _____

Part Two: An essential part of a Central Service technician's job is to understand the rationale (reason) behind infection control protocols (requirements). Use the space provided below under each protocol to explain the rationale (reason why) each is important.

1. Central Service technicians change from their street clothes into clean attire before entering their work area.

    _____

    _____

    _____

2. Before beginning work, Central Service technicians remove jewelry.

    _____

    _____

    _____

3. Central Service technicians wear personal protective equipment in the decontamination area.

    _____

    _____

    _____

4. Food and beverages are not allowed in Central Service work areas.

    _____

    _____

    _____

5. Floors in the Central Service department should be wet mopped daily; they should never be swept or dust mopped.

    _____

    _____

    _____

Part Three: List the six elements in the chain of infection.

1. _____

2. _____

3. _____

4. _____

5. _____

6. _____

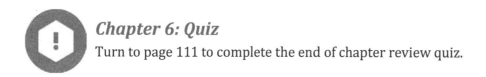

Chapter 6: Quiz
Turn to page 111 to complete the end of chapter review quiz.

Chapter 7

Decontamination: Point-of-Use Preparation and Transport

 ## *Learning Objectives*

As a result of successfully completing this chapter, users will be able to:

1. Review the four main goals of soiled item preparation and transport

2. Identify the sources of contaminated items

3. Explain point-of-use preparation procedures

4. Review basic procedures to transport soiled items from user areas to the Central Service decontamination area

5. Discuss safety guidelines for transporting soiled items to the Central Service decontamination area

6. Identify basic sources for education and training information applicable to the transport of contaminated items

 ## *Reading Assignment*

Read Chapter 7 in the *Central Service Technical Manual, Eighth Edition.*

Chapter 7: Practice Exercises

Use the list of terms below to complete each statement (there will be more word selections than needed and some may be used more than once).

Biofilm	Decontamination	Moist
Biohazard	End of procedure	Open
Cleaned	End user	Point-of-use
Cleaning	Equipment area	Separated
Closed	Gross soil	Soiled
Contaminated	Hard sided	Surgery
Decontaminated	Identified	Wire

1. The _____ department is the major source of soiled items received by the Central Service department.

2. Containers dedicated to the transport of small quantities of soiled instruments should be clearly marked with a _____ label.

3. When instruments are prepared for transport to the decontamination area it is important to keep them _____.

4. Tissue, body fat, blood and other bodily substances are examples of _____.

5. Disposable sharp items should be removed at the point of use and placed in a _____ container labeled _____.

6. Point-of-use preparation of soiled items begins the _____ process.

7. Disposable items and linen should be removed at _____.

8. Soiled instruments should be transported in a _____ container or cart.

9. Reusable sharps should be _____ from other instruments and placed in a separate container so they can be _____ easily.

10. Containers and carts used to transport contaminated items should NOT be used to transport clean items unless they have been thoroughly _____ between uses.

Chapter 7: Quiz

Turn to page 113 to complete the end of chapter review quiz.

Chapter 8
Cleaning and Decontamination

Learning Objectives

As a result of successfully completing this chapter, users will be able to:

1. Define cleaning and identify challenges to cleaning medical devices
2. Discuss the purpose and set up of the decontamination area
3. Identify the importance of personal protective equipment and standard precautions
4. Explain the role of common cleaning tools
5. Discuss mechanical cleaners
6. Discuss the use of chemicals in the decontamination area
7. List steps in the cleaning process
8. Explain manual cleaning processes

Reading Assignment

Read Chapter 8 in the *Central Service Technical Manual, Eighth Edition.*

Chapter 8: Practice Exercises

On the following page, indicate whether each statement is true or false.

1. Instruments with lumens should always be soaked in a vertical position and should not be soaked in a horizontal position.
    a. True
    b. False

2. The mechanical process by which an ultrasonic cleaner works is called cavitation.
    a. True
    b. False

3. To prevent aerosols, items should be brushed below the surface of the water.
    a. True
    b. False

4. Automatic washers clean using a spray-force action called impingement.
    a. True
    b. False

5. Instruments received from surgery and tagged for repair do not need to be cleaned until they come back from repair.
    a. True
    b. False

6. Powered surgical instruments should be cleaned using a mechanical cleaning process.
    a. True
    b. False

7. There are currently no methods available to verify cleaning process outcomes.
    a. True
    b. False

8. All sonic cleaners have a decontamination cycle.
    a. True
    b. False

9. Horizontal work surfaces in the decontamination area should be cleaned and disinfected once per day.
    a. True
    b. False

10. Because of the cavitation and impingement action of mechanical cleaners, there is no need to pre-clean items that will be processed in a mechanical cleaner.
    a. True
    b. False

Chapter 8: Quiz
Turn to page 115 to complete the end of chapter review quiz.

PROGRESS TEST TWO

Turn to page 183 to complete **Progress Test Two** before continuing on to Chapter 9.

Chapter 9
Disinfection

Learning Objectives

As a result of successfully completing this chapter, users will be able to:

1. Define the term disinfection and explain how disinfection differs from sterilization

2. Explain disinfection levels as identified in the Spaulding Classification System:
   - Low-level disinfection
   - Intermediate-level disinfection
   - High-level disinfection

3. Provide basic information about the types of disinfectants commonly used in healthcare facilities:
   - Quaternary ammonium compounds
   - Alcohol
   - Phenolics
   - Chlorine
   - Iodophors
   - Glutaraldehyde
   - Ortho-phthalaldehyde
   - Hydrogen peroxide
   - Peracetic acid

4. Identify good work practices for manual disinfection processes

5. Discuss automated equipment utilized for disinfection, and good work practices for working with automated disinfection processes

6. Explain disinfection quality assurance practices

Reading Assignment

Read Chapter 9 in the *Central Service Technical Manual, Eighth Edition.*

Chapter 9: Practice Exercises

Part One: Matching

Match the word below with the correct description (there will be more word selections than needed).

a. Antiseptic
b. Disinfectant
c. Bactericidal
d. Thermal disinfection
e. Sterilization
f. Ortho-phthalaldehyde
g. Alcohol

h. Wet contact time
i. Disinfectant holding time
j. Disinfection
k. Each use
l. Daily
m. Air bubbles
n. Phenolic
o. Microorganisms

___ 1. The use of heat to kill all microorganisms except spores.

___ 2. A chemical which kills most pathogenic organisms, but does not kill spores.

___ 3. A solution which inhibits the growth of bacteria usually used topically and only on animate objects.

___ 4. The length of time an item must remain wet with a disinfectant.

___ 5. The destruction of nearly all pathogenic microorganisms on an inanimate surface.

___ 6. Relating to the destruction of bacteria.

___ 7. The frequency the concentration level of a high-level disinfectant must be tested.

___ 8. A process by which all forms of microbial life are destroyed.

___ 9. Minimum effective concentration testing is required when using this disinfectant.

___ 10. When manually disinfecting lumens, care should be taken to ensure there are no _____present inside the lumens.

Part Two: Name the Disinfectant
Use the clues below to identify the type of disinfectant being described.

1. This low-level disinfectant is often used in environmental sanitation such as on floors, walls and furniture. It is incompatible with soaps. Its concentration may be diminished by some materials such as cotton, wool, filter paper and charcoal.

    It is: _____

2. This high-level disinfectant is used for semi-critical devices such as endoscopes. Once it is activated (mixed) it must be checked routinely using test strips to ensure its concentration. Because of its fumes employees who work with it must follow specific Occupational Safety and Health Administration guidelines for safety.

    It is: _____

3. This common disinfectant has been in use for several years. It is often used to disinfect equipment. It is inactivated by organic soil. In order to achieve a reasonable level of disinfection, it must remain in wet contact with the item being disinfected for at least five minutes; this can be a problem because it evaporates quickly.

    It is: _____

4. This intermediate-level disinfectant is a member of the halogen disinfectant family. Although it may be found in Central Service decontamination areas, it is not recommended for use on instruments because of its corrosive qualities.

    It is: _____

Chapter 9: Quiz

Turn to page 117 to complete the end of chapter review quiz.

Chapter 10
Surgical Instrumentation

Learning Objectives

As a result of successfully completing this chapter, users will be able to:

1. Discuss the importance of surgical instruments and the role of the Central Service technician in instrument care and handling

2. Review basic steps in the surgical instrument manufacturing process

3. Define basic categories of surgical instruments based upon their functions and identify the points of inspection, anatomy and procedures to measure the following types of instruments:
    *   Hemostatic forceps
    *   Needle holders
    *   Tissue forceps
    *   Dressing forceps
    *   Retractors
    *   Scissors
    *   Suction devices
    *   Single- and double-action rongeurs
    *   Kerrison/laminectomy rongeurs
    *   Nail nippers
    *   Graves and Pederson vaginal speculums

4. Identify solutions that can damage stainless steel instruments

5. Explain procedures to test instruments for sharpness and to identify (mark) them

6. Emphasize the importance of instrument lubrication and review tray assembly safeguards

Reading Assignment

Read Chapter 10 in the *Central Service Technical Manual, Eighth Edition.*

Chapter 10: Practice Exercises

Part One: Matching

Match the term below with the correct description (there will be more word selections than needed).

a. Osteotomes   f. Saline   k. Box locks
b. Rongeurs   g. Forceps   l. Gelpi
c. Martensitic   h. Scissors   m. Richardson
d. Passivation   i. Chisels   n. Tungsten carbide
e. Ratchet   j. Austenitic   o. Black

___ 1. A self-retaining retractor.

___ 2. Part that locks the handles in place on a ring-handled surgical instrument.

___ 3. Surgical instruments used to cut away at bone and tissue.

___ 4. A chemical process applied during instrument manufacture that provides a corrosion-resistant finish.

___ 5. Also known as 400 series stainless steel, this metal used in surgical instrument manufacturing can be heat hardened.

___ 6. Surgical instruments used to cut, incise or dissect tissue.

___ 7. Commonly found in the Operating Room, this can damage instruments with prolonged exposure.

___ 8. Surgical instruments used to grasp.

___ 9. Where the two parts of a ring-handled instrument meet and pivot.

___ 10. Inserts for needle holders are frequently made of this metal.

Part Two: True or False

Indicate whether each of the following statements is true or false.

1. Tungsten carbide scissors blades hold a sharp edge longer than stainless steel blades.
   a. True
   b. False

2. Tissue forceps have teeth and dressing forceps have serrations.
   a. True
   b. False

3. Double-action rongeurs should be tested for sharpness using tissue paper.
   a. True
   b. False

4. Laser etching is an acceptable method for marking instruments.
   a. True
   b. False

5. Because they are mild cleaners, dish soaps are the cleaners of choice for surgical instruments.
   a. True
   b. False

Part Three: Labeling

Label the parts of this instrument.

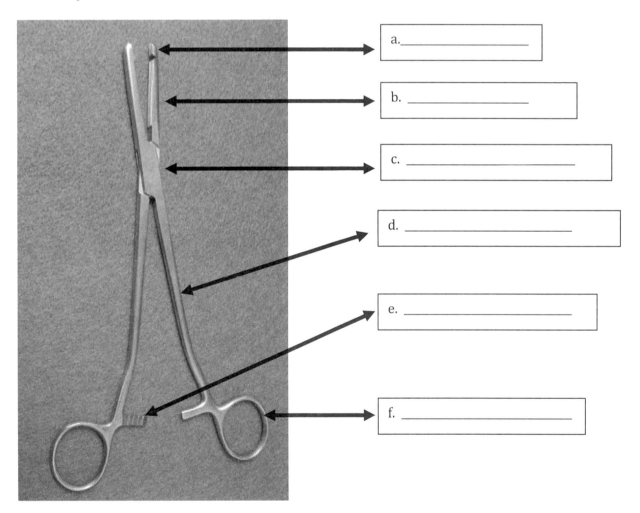

a._____

b. _____

c. _____

d. _____

e. _____

f. _____

Chapter 10: Quiz

Turn to page 119 to complete the end of chapter review quiz.

Chapter 11
Complex Surgical Instruments

 ## *Learning Objectives*

As a result of successfully completing this chapter, users will be able to:

1. Provide an overview of and discuss procedures to care for and effectively process powered surgical instruments

2. Explain important basic concerns when handling and processing endoscopic instruments

3. Discuss detailed information about rigid and flexible endoscopes and their accessories

4. Review general processing and inspection requirements for endoscopes and accessories

5. Identify infection prevention concerns regarding endoscopes and loaner instrumentation

6. Identify basic protocols important for each step in the loaner instrumentation process

 ## *Reading Assignment*

Read Chapter 11 in the *Central Service Technical Manual, Eighth Edition.*

 ## *Chapter 11: Practice Exercises*

Part One: Match the powered surgical instrument with its use.

a. Dermatome/dermabraider
b. Cebatome
c. Sternal saw

d. Dental drill
e. Micro drill
f. Saw

___ 1.   Used to repair and reconstruct teeth and jawbones.

___ 2.   Used in ear surgery and for driving very small wires through bone.

___ 3.   Used in open heart surgery.

___ 4.   Used to remove cement.

___ 5.   Used to harvest skin grafts and reshape skin surfaces.

___ 6.   Used to perform specific cutting actions such as reciprocating or oscillating.

Part Two: On the following page, match the endoscope with its use.

a.	Bronchoscope	c.	Gastroscope	e.	Colonoscope
b.	Cystoscope	d.	Sigmoidoscope		

___ 1. Allows for visual inspection of the lower part of the large intestine.

___ 2. Allows for visual inspection of the upper digestive tract.

___ 3. Used to visualize the urethra and bladder.

___ 4. Used to visualize the tracheobronchial tree.

___ 5. Used to visualize the entire large intestine.

Part Three: Indicate whether each of the following statements is true or false.

1. Leak testing should be performed on each flexible endoscope on an annual basis.
    a. True
    b. False

2. Loaner instrument trays that are received sterile from other facilities do not need to be decontaminated and re-sterilized before use.
    a. True
    b. False

3. Endoscope channels should be cleaned and then left moist for storage.
    a. True
    b. False

4. Powered surgical instruments have one of three power sources: electricity, air or battery.
    a. True
    b. False

5. Modern powered surgical instruments can be immersed.
    a. True
    b. False

6. Laparoscopic instrument insulation failure can cause burns.
    a. True
    b. False

7. The purpose of a decontamination battery is to protect powered surgical instruments from fluid invasion.
    a. True
    b. False

8. Dental drills are used to remove cement.
    a. True
    b. False

9. Automatic endoscope reprocessors are not recommended for flexible endoscopes.
    a. True
    b. False

Chapter 11: Quiz

Turn to page 121 to complete the end of chapter review quiz.

Chapter 12
Assembly and Packaging

Learning Objectives

As a result of successfully completing this chapter, users will be able to:

1. Explain the set up and function of the assembly area

2. Review basic procedures to prepare pack contents for packaging

3. Explain the basic objectives of the packaging process and review basic selection factors for materials to be used with specific sterilization methods

4. Provide an overview of reusable packaging materials

5. Provide an overview of disposable packaging materials

6. Discuss basic package closure methods

7. Review general packaging concepts:
   - Package labeling
   - Special concerns
   - Sterility maintenance

Reading Assignment

Read Chapter 12 in the *Central Service Technical Manual, Eighth Edition.*

Chapter 12: Practice Exercises

Match the term below with the correct description (there will be more word selections than needed).

a. Paper
b. Plastic
c. U.S. Food and Drug Administration
d. Environmental Protection Agency
e. Reusable
f. Disposable
g. Four hours
h. Two hours

i. Paper/plastic combinations
j. Indicator tapes
k. Paperclips
l. Sequential
m. Simultaneous
n. Square fold
o. Envelope fold
p. Spunbond polyolefin-plastic combinations

___ 1. An acceptable method of package closure that is also used as an external indicator.

___ 2. Minimum amount of time that packaging materials should be held at room temperature and at 30% to 70% relative humidity before sterilization.

___ 3. Flat wrapping technique that applies one wrap on top of another to create a package within a package.

___ 4. Government agency that regulates sterilization packaging materials.

___ 5. This type of packaging contains no cellulosic materials and would be used to package small items for low-temperature sterilization.

___ 6. This type of packaging can be used in steam and ethylene oxide sterilization but is not recommended for other types of sterilization.

___ 7. When using paper/plastic pouches, package content information should be written on this side of the pouch.

___ 8. This is NOT an acceptable method of package closure.

___ 9. Muslin is an example of this type of packaging material.

___ 10. The wrapping technique most commonly used for small packs and most trays.

Chapter 12: Quiz

Turn to page 123 to complete the end of chapter review quiz.

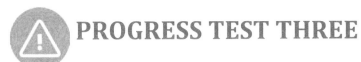

PROGRESS TEST THREE

Turn to page 189 to complete **Progress Test Three** before continuing on to Chapter 13.

Chapter 13
Point-of-Use Processing

Learning Objectives

As a result of successfully completing this chapter, users will be able to:

1. Define the term Immediate Use Steam Sterilization and review the industry standards

2. Describe point-of-use processing and examine its requirements

3. Explain the basic procedures necessary to safely perform Immediate Use Steam Sterilization

4. Discuss point-of-use processing of heat-sensitive medical devices

Reading Assignment

Read Chapter 13 in the *Central Service Technical Manual, Eighth Edition.*

Chapter 13: Practice Exercises

Indicate whether each of the following statements is true or false.

1. Sterilization documentation is not required for items that are steam sterilized for immediate use.
    a. True
    b. False

2. Instruments must be cleaned before being sterilized for immediate use.
    a. True
    b. False

3. Personal protective equipment is not required when cleaning items for Immediate Use Steam Sterilization.
    a. True
    b. False

4. The sterilization method of choice for single-use items is Immediate Use Steam Sterilization.
    a. True
    b. False

5. It is recommended to use Immediate Use Steam Sterilization to sterilize instruments contaminated with Creutzfeldt-Jakob disease after the procedure has been completed.
    a. True
    b. False

6. Immediate Use Steam Sterilization was developed to process items when the facility does not have enough instruments to perform the surgery.
    a. True
    b. False

7. To sterilize items using steam, the item's manufacturer instructions must state the item can be sterilized using an immediate use steam sterilization cycle.
    a. True
    b. False

8. When processing items for immediate use, items do not need to be disassembled prior to cleaning.
    a. True
    b. False

9. When using low-temperature methods for sterilization or disinfection of items at the point of use, item preparation is not as critical as when preparing items for terminal sterilization.
    a. True
    b. False

10. All items sterilized or high-level disinfected at the point of use must be carefully monitored and logged.
    a. True
    b. False

Chapter 13: Quiz

Turn to page 125 to complete the end of chapter review quiz.

Chapter 14
High-Temperature Sterilization

Learning Objectives

As a result of successfully completing this chapter, users will be able to:

1. Discuss factors that impact the effectiveness of sterilization
2. Discuss the advantages of steam sterilization
3. Explain the anatomy of a steam sterilizer and identify the function of each major component
4. Provide basic information about the types of steam sterilizers
5. Explain basic information about steam sterilizer cycles
6. Describe the conditions necessary for an effective steam sterilization process
7. Explain basic work practices for steam sterilization
8. Review sterilization process indicators and explain the need for quality control

Reading Assignment

Read Chapter 14 in the *Central Service Technical Manual, Eighth Edition.*

Chapter 14: Practice Exercises

Fill in the blanks using words from the list on the following page (there will be more word selections than needed).

Printer pens
Convection
Condensate
Bioburden
Thermostatic trap
Gravity
Dynamic air removal
Pre-vacuum
Jacket
Dry
Gasket

Chamber drain
Wet
Bacillus atrophaeus
Geobacillus stearothermophilus
Cleaning
Charts and printouts
Contact
Verification
Bowie-Dick test
Exposure
Chemical integrator

1. The interior chamber walls of the sterilizer are heated by steam in the _____ of the sterilizer.

2. The _____ is designed to maintain a tight seal that prevents steam from escaping the chamber of a sterilizer.

3. The _____ is located in the floor of the steam sterilizer.

4. The portion of the steam sterilizer that measures steam temperature and automatically controls the flow of air and condensate from the sterilizer chamber is the

   _____.

5. _____ provide a written record of sterilizer cycle activities.

6. _____ sterilizers remove air from the chamber by steam forcing the cooler air in the chamber out through the drain.

7. The most frequent cause for sterilization failure is lack of steam _____.

8. Inadequate _____ time at the correct elevated temperature is a reason for sterilization failure.

9. Another name for superheated steam is _____ steam.

10. Placing warm sterilized packages on cool surfaces will cause _____ to form.

Chapter 14: Quiz

Turn to page 127 to complete the end of chapter review quiz.

Chapter 15
Low-Temperature Sterilization

Learning Objectives

As a result of successfully completing this chapter, users will be able to:

1. Discuss basic requirements important for all low-temperature sterilization systems

2. Explain specific requirements for low-temperature sterilization methods commonly used by healthcare facilities:
   - Ethylene oxide
   - Hydrogen peroxide
   - Ozone

3. Review important parameters of the low-temperature sterilization methods

Reading Assignment

Read Chapter 15 in the *Central Service Technical Manual, Eighth Edition.*

Chapter 15: Practice Exercises

Use the list of terms below to complete each statement on the following page (there will be more word selections than needed).

Ozone
Ethylene oxide
4.5 hours
Oxygen
2.5 hours
Eight hours

Bacillus atrophaeus
Geobacillus stearothermophilus
Ethylene glycol
Sterility assurance level
Occupational Safety and Health Administration
U.S. Food and Drug Administration

1. _____is a byproduct of ozone sterilization.

2. The_____ method of low-temperature sterilization uses gas cartridges for a sterilant.

3. The probability of a viable microorganism being present on an item after sterilization is the _____.

4. The bacterial spore used to test ethylene oxide sterilization cycles is

   _____.

5. Cycle time for items sterilized using ozone sterilization is_____.

6. An aeration time of _____ at 140⁰ F is recommended for items sterilized with ethylene oxide.

7. _____ is a bacterial spore used to test hydrogen peroxide sterilization cycles.

8. Exposure time for items sterilized using ethylene oxide sterilization is

   _____.

9. _____sets exposure standards for chemical sterilants.

10. _____recommends that sterilants be rigorously tested before being marketed.

Chapter 15: Quiz

Turn to page 131 to complete the end of chapter review quiz.

Chapter 16
Sterile Storage and Transport

Learning Objectives

As a result of successfully completing this chapter, users will be able to:

1. Review basic sterile storage considerations
2. Describe basic types of sterile storage shelving
3. Identify procedures for moving sterile items into storage
4. Explain the concept of event-related sterility
5. Discuss basic storage guidelines
6. Discuss other sterile storage and transport concerns:
   - Basic procedures for cleaning sterile storage areas
   - Sterile storage personnel
   - Transporting sterile items
   - Transportation guidelines

Reading Assignment

Read Chapter 16 in the *Central Service Technical Manual, Eighth Edition.*

Chapter 16: Practice Exercises

Use the list of terms below to complete each statement (there will be more word selections than needed).

a. Positive
b. 75 or lower
c. Gasket
d. Reusable
e. Disposable
f. 30% to 60%
g. Filter
h. 8 to 10

i. Should
j. Should not
k. 18
l. Barrier packaging
m. Negative
n. Less than 70%
o. Bottom
p. First in, first out

___ 1. _____is a method of stock rotation which ensures that older items are used first.

___ 2. Air flow in the sterile storage area should be _____.

___ 3. Packaging that prevents microorganisms from entering the packages and allows aseptic opening is called_____.

___ 4. Humidity in the sterile storage area should be _____.

___ 5. Temperature in the sterile storage area should be_____.

___ 6. The _____ shelf of storage carts should be solid.

___ 7. Items _____ be used after the manufacturer's expiration date as long as the package integrity is still intact.

___ 8. Stacking rigid containers too high can cause _____ damage.

___ 9. Items should be stored at least _____ inches below sprinkler heads.

___ 10. When transporting sterile items in a dedicated clean lift they _____ be contained.

Chapter 16: Quiz

Turn to page 133 to complete the end of chapter review quiz.

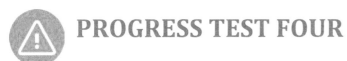

PROGRESS TEST FOUR

Turn to page 197 to complete **Progress Test Four** before continuing on to Chapter 17.

Chapter 17
Monitoring and Recordkeeping for Central Service

Learning Objectives

As a result of successfully completing this chapter, users will be able to:

1. Discuss the importance of monitoring work areas and processes within the Central Service department

2. Discuss the importance of recordkeeping

3. Explain the types of monitoring needed in each area of the Central Service department

4. Explain the need for monitoring and review of the sterilization process indicators that help assure quality control:
   - Need for monitoring
   - Chemical indicators
   - Sterilization load control information
   - Physical and mechanical monitors
   - Biological indicators
   - Bowie-Dick tests

5. Discuss the importance of employee training and continuing education records

Reading Assignment

Read Chapter 17 in the *Central Service Technical Manual, Eighth Edition.*

Chapter 17: Practice Exercises

Use the list of terms below to complete each statement (there will be more word selections than needed).

a. Court
b. Continuing education records
c. Load (lot) control label
d. Temperature and humidity
e. Cavitation
f. External indicator
g. Negative
h. Impingement
i. Leak test

j. Interviews
k. Sterilizer control log
l. Production number
m. Julian date
n. Positive
o. Scale
p. Competency
q. Biological test
r. Biological indicator process challenge devices

___ 1. The _____ is the dating system that uses the number of days that have elapsed in the year.

___ 2. Keeping records accurate and complete is important because they are used during The Joint Commission and Centers for Medicare and Medicaid Services surveys, but may also be used in _____.

___ 3. _____records are kept to provide evidence that an employee has kept current and is aware of new best practices.

___ 4. A _____ should be run in every sterilizer load that contains implants.

___ 5. Recording _____ is an example of formal monitoring.

___ 6. Label that contains the date, sterilizer identification and sterilizer cycle number is called a _____.

___ 7. _____ are used to help determine where employees excel or where they may need additional training.

___ 8. Ultrasonic cleaners clean by a process called _____.

___ 9. A test performed to help ensure there are no air leaks in a steam sterilizer is called a _____.

___ 10. If there is no bacterial growth in a biological indicator after sterilization and incubation it is called a _____ test.

Chapter 17: Quiz

Turn to page 135 to complete the end of chapter review quiz.

Chapter 18
Quality Assurance

Learning Objectives

As a result of successfully completing this chapter, users will be able to:

1. Define quality in the context of Central Service operations

2. Describe the components of a Central Service quality program

3. Explain the basics of failure mode and effects analysis and root cause analysis

4. Discuss common quality programs:
   - Total quality improvement
   - Continuous quality improvement
   - Total quality management
   - Six Sigma and Lean
   - Other quality programs and standards

5. Review quality procedures in the Central Service department

Reading Assignment

Read Chapter 18 in the *Central Service Technical Manual, Eighth Edition.*

Chapter 18: Practice Exercises

Recall key facts about quality assurance by completing each sentence below.

1. Nurses, physicians and other professionals working in a healthcare facility are

    _____ customers of Central Service.

2. An activity designed to identify and resolve work task-related problems is called

    _____ .

3. The consistent delivery of products and services according to established standards is called

    _____.

4. The _____ must be the center of every quality concern.

5. A process that looks backwards at an event to help prevent it from reoccurring is called a

    _____.

6. The quality process that uses DMADV/DMAIC to improve processes is called

    _____ .

7. _____ is an international standard used by participating organizations to help assure that they consistently deliver quality services and products.

8. The act of granting authority to employees to make decisions within their areas of responsibility is called

    _____.

9. A series of work activities which produce a product or service is called a

    _____.

10. An unexpected occurrence involving death, serious physical or psychological injury or the risk thereof is called a

    _____.

Chapter 18: Quiz

Turn to page 137 to complete the end of chapter review quiz.

Chapter 19
Managing Inventory within the Central Service Department

Learning Objectives

As a result of successfully completing this chapter, users will be able to:

1. Explain the importance of inventory management in the healthcare facility

2. Define the role of Central Service technicians as it relates to inventory management

3. Explain basic inventory terms used in healthcare facilities

4. Explain the cycle of consumable items

5. Discuss the partnership between Central Service and Materiel Management

6. Describe guidelines for handling commercially sterilized packages

7. Describe common inventory replenishment systems
    - Periodic automatic replenishment-level systems
    - Automated supply replenishment systems
    - Exchange cart systems
    - Requisition systems
    - Case cart systems
    - STAT orders

8. Discuss the role of healthcare facilities in sustainability efforts and the reduction of waste

Reading Assignment

Read Chapter 19 in the *Central Service Technical Manual, Eighth Edition.*

Chapter 19: Practice Exercises

Part One: Terminology

Use the list of terms below to complete each statement (there will be more word selections than needed).

Consumable inventory   STAT
Reusable inventory   Sustainability
Distribution   Asset
Case cart   Capital

1. When items are needed immediately (at once) Central Service technicians

   may receive a _____ order.

2. Something of value that is owned by an organization or person is called an

   _____.

3. Detergents, sterilization quality assurance products and other items that
   are purchased, used up and replaced are called

   _____.

4. Sterilizers, mechanical washers and other expensive items are examples

   of _____ equipment.

5. The act of moving supplies throughout the facility is called _____.

6. Process designed to reduce harm to the environment is called _____.

Part Two: Name the system

Use the clues below to identify the type of system being described.

1. This inventory replenishment system uses identical carts filled with supplies. One
   cart is dispensed to the user unit and the second cart is kept on standby. Then at a
   specified time, the second (full) cart is taken to the user unit to replace the used one.
   The used cart is taken to the storage area, restocked and held until the next
   scheduled replacement time.

   Name the system: _____

2. This inventory system is usually used to manage instruments and supplies for individual surgical procedures. A cart filled with instruments and supplies is assembled for each specific procedure and delivered to the user unit, usually the Operating Room.

   Name the system: _____

3. In this system needed items are requested by the user unit, the order is received and filled from a central storage location. The requested items are then delivered to the requesting (user) unit.

   Name the system: _____

4. In this system a predetermined quantity of supplies is stored on the user unit. Central Service/Materiel Management staff inventory the supply stock on the user unit and replenish used supplies to ensure that stock levels are returned to the predetermined quantities.

   Name the system: _____

5. This system is a computerized system that allows clinical staff to obtain patient items from a storage unit on the user unit. When the item is removed the clinical staff keys in a code or uses a scan to account for the items they are removing. That data is compiled by the computer and at an established time, an order is generated to restock the storage unit.

   Name the system: _____

Part Three: Identification

Identify each symbol below.

1. _____

2. _____

3. _____

4. _____

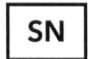

5. _____

6. _____

 Chapter 19: Quiz
Turn to page 139 to complete the end of chapter review quiz.

Chapter 20
The Role of Central Service in Ancillary Department Support

Learning Objectives

As a result of successfully completing this chapter, users will be able to:

1. Discuss the role that the Central Service department plays in supporting ancillary departments

2. Discuss strategies for managing patient care equipment

3. Explain the importance of communication and coordination as it relates to ancillary support

Reading Assignment

Read Chapter 20 in the *Central Service Technical Manual, Eighth Edition.*

Chapter 20: Practice Exercises

Part One: Matching

Match the term below with the correct description (there will be more word selections than needed).

a. Defibrillator
b. Foot pump
c. Sequential compression device
d. Infusion pump
e. Hypothermia unit
f. Patient-controlled analgesia
g. Biomedical engineering
h. Wound vacuum assisted closure therapy
i. Preventive maintenance
j. Repair
k. Central Service
l. Continuous passive range of pump motion device

___ 1. The department that checks patient care equipment for safety and function.

___ 2. Allows the patient to self-administer pain medication.

___ 3. Applies a brief electroshock to restore the rhythm of the heart.

___ 4. Artificially stimulates the venous plantar plexus to increase circulation in bed-ridden patients.

___ 5. This device moves joints after surgery or trauma.

___ 6. This unit is used to raise or lower body temperature.

Part Two: Indicate whether each of the following statements is true or false.

1. Manufacturers sometimes loan equipment to facilities at no cost if the facility agrees to purchase disposable equipment components from the manufacturer.
    a. True
    b. False

2. A gastric suction unit is used to suction liquids from oral and nasal cavities.
    a. True
    b. False

3. Both Biomedical technicians and Central Service technicians are qualified to repair patient care equipment.
    a. True
    b. False

4. Used equipment that is not visibly soiled may be returned to the clean equipment storage area without undergoing a decontamination process.
    a. True
    b. False

Chapter 20: Quiz

Turn to page 141 to complete the end of chapter review quiz.

PROGRESS TEST FIVE

Turn to page 209 to complete **Progress Test Five** before continuing on to Chapter 21.

Chapter 21

The Role of Information Technology in Central Service

Learning Objectives

As a result of successfully completing this chapter, users will be able to:

1. Provide an overview of the use of information management systems in Central Service departments

2. Discuss the use of computers and information systems to support activities within the healthcare facility and Central Service department

3. Recognize that tracking systems enhance Central Service operations

4. Explain why tracking systems must address the specific needs of the healthcare facility and Central Service department

5. Review some features of available instrument and equipment tracking systems

Reading Assignment

Read Chapter 21 in the *Central Service Technical Manual, Eighth Edition.*

Chapter 21: Practice Exercises

Complete the following sections.

1. List six reasons why it is important for the Central Service department to track items.

   _____

   _____

   _____

   _____

   _____

   _____

2. Interfaced, cloud based or turnkey: which of these terms means systems communicate with each other?

   _____

3. Name two types of tracking systems.

   _____

   _____

4. List three things a basic instrument and equipment tracking system can track.

   _____

   _____

   _____

Chapter 21: Quiz

Turn to page 145 to complete the end of chapter review quiz.

Chapter 22
Safety and Risk Management for Central Service

Learning Objectives

As a result of successfully completing this chapter, users will be able to:

1. Explain the importance of safety and risk management in the Central Service department

2. Review three common workplace hazards: fire, hazardous substances and bloodborne pathogens

3. Explain the importance of ergonomics and health awareness for Central Service technicians

4. Discuss common safety hazards applicable to Central Service functions and work areas, and explain how employee injuries can be prevented

5. Describe special safety precautions for handling ethylene oxide

6. Discuss the basics of internal and external disaster plans for a healthcare facility

7. Review procedures to report employee accidents and injuries

8. Explain the importance of education and reporting in a Central Service safety and risk management system

Reading Assignment

Read Chapter 22 in the *Central Service Technical Manual, Eighth Edition.*

Chapter 22: Practice Exercises

Part One: Fill in the blanks.

1. The three types of hazards found in the Central Service department are

   _____, _____ and _____.

2. The methods used to assess the risks of a specific activity, and to develop a program to reduce losses from exposure to those risks is called

   _____.

3. You would find physical data relating to a chemical on the _____.

4. Occupational Safety and Health Administration has established permissible exposure limits for many chemicals like hydrogen peroxide and ozone as

   _____.

5. The three elements that make up the fire triangle are _____,

   _____ and _____.

Part Two: Indicate whether each of the following statements is true or false.

1. If an injury seems insignificant, there is no need to report it.
   a. True
   b. False

2. Preparation and sterilization areas pose no risk of injury to Central Service technicians.
   a. True
   b. False

3. Gas cylinder regulators are interchangeable between different types of gases.
   a. True
   b. False

4. Loss of the Central Service department's water supply would be an example of an internal disaster.
   a. True
   b. False

5. Part of a facilities employee training plan should include emergency spill procedures and how to read safety data sheets.
   a. True
   b. False

Part Three: Which of the following hazards would you commonly find in the Central Service department? Check all that apply.

___	Asbestos	___	Needlesticks and punctures
___	Ethylene oxide	___	Freons
___	Radiation	___	Paints and solvents
___	Mercury	___	Bloodborne pathogens
___	Infectious agents	___	Ergonomic stressors
___	Boiler compounds	___	Burns
___	Chemicals	___	Falls
___	Adhesives	___	Chemical fixers and developer

Chapter 22: Quiz
Turn to page 147 to complete the end of chapter review quiz.

Chapter 23
Success through Communication

Learning Objectives

As a result of successfully completing this chapter, users will be able to:

1. Explain why Central Service technicians must use effective communication and human relations skills

2. Define the term "professionalism," list traits of professional Central Service technicians and describe their fundamental beliefs and behaviors

3. Describe behaviors that can impact success on the job

4. Use basic tactics of effective communication in the workplace

5. Practice procedures to enhance and maintain effective working relationships

6. Discuss tactics to improve teamwork

7. Define the term "diversity" and explain why it is important

8. Practice basic customer service skills and utilize tactics to appropriately handle customer complaints

9. Review common workplace communication issues

Reading Assignment

Read Chapter 23 in the *Central Service Technical Manual, Eighth Edition.*

Chapter 23: Practice Exercises

Match the term with the correct description below.

a. Communication
b. Human relations
c. Ethical behavior
d. Attitude
e. Legal behavior
f. Feedback

g. Coaching
h. Mentoring
i. Diversity
j. Service recovery
k. Teamwork
l. Professionalism

___ 1. The sequence of steps used to address customer complaints.

___ 2. Positive reinforcement used to encourage employees to follow proper work practices and negative reinforcement to discourage inappropriate work practices.

___ 3. This communication process occurs when the listener asks a question, repeats information or otherwise helps the speaker to know if the message has been correctly received.

___ 4. Behavior relating to what is right or wrong relative to the standards of conduct for a profession.

___ 5. The process of transmitting information and understanding from one person to another by use of words and non-verbal expressions such as body language.

___ 6. The broad range of human characteristics and dimensions which impact an employee's values, opportunities and perceptions of themselves and others at work.

Chapter 23: Quiz

Turn to page 149 to complete the end of chapter review quiz.

Chapter 24
Personal and Professional Development for Central Service

Learning Objectives

As a result of successfully completing this chapter, users will be able to:

1. Explain the meaning of personal development and how it can impact a career in the Central Service department

2. List possible Central Service career paths

3. Review strategies for professional goal setting

4. Discuss strategies to enhance professional skills and expertise

5. Discuss resumé development

6. Review the interview process

7. Discuss promotions

Reading Assignment

Read Chapter 24 in the *Central Service Technical Manual, Eighth Edition.*

Chapter 24: Practice Exercises

Use the list of terms below to complete each statement (there will be more word selections than needed).

a. Professional development
b. Resources
c. Personal development
d. Subordinate
e. Network
f. Interview
g. Public speaking

h. Closed-ended
i. Conferences
j. Resumé
k. Writing skills
l. Open-ended
m. Certification
n. Online

___ 1. Developing professional resources in the field of Central Service can

provide a _____ to share information.

___ 2. Attending educational _____ is one way to help achieve career goals.

___ 3. One of the most important factors in attaining goals is finding the right

_____.

___ 4. _____ identifies and develops talent as well as improves employability.

___ 5. "Do you like your job?" is an example of a/an _____ question.

___ 6. A _____ is a compilation of skills, education and accomplishments.

Chapter 24: Quiz

Turn to page 151 to complete the end of chapter review quiz.

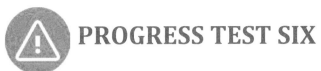

PROGRESS TEST SIX

Turn to page 225 to complete **Progress Test Six.**

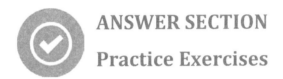

ANSWER SECTION

Practice Exercises

Chapter 1: Introduction to Central Service Practice Exercises page reference

1. Since Central Service technicians do not handle money, ethics considerations do not apply to them.
    b. *False*   *(17)*

2. Central Service technicians practice resource management when they control costs and reduce waste.
    a. *True*   *(18)*

3. Central Service technicians must be able to identify approximately 100 surgical instruments in order to be proficient in their job.
    b. *False*   *(11)*

4. Central Service technicians must be able to adapt to change.
    a. *True*   *(16)*

5. Because all Central Service departments are structured alike, healthcare facilities use one standard job description for all Central Service technicians.
    b. *False*   *(18)*

6. Career growth and progression is virtually nonexistent for Central Service technicians.
    b. *False*   *(19)*

7. Departments that perform Central Service functions may go by other names at different facilities; for example, Sterile Processing and Distribution or Surgical Supply.
    a. *True*   *(10)*

8. Central Service workflow can be divided into the handling of three categories of items: soiled items, clean items and sterile items.
    a. *True*   *(9)*

9. The use of good verbal communication skills is the most important and most used skill for Central Service technicians to provide or obtain information.
    b. *False*   *(15)*

10. Since modern Central Service departments are virtually risk free, Central Service technicians need not be concerned with safety practices.
    b. *False*   *(17)*

Chapter 2: Medical Terminology for Central Service Technicians Practice Exercises

Part One:

1. The prefix *hyper-* means *above, excessive* while the prefix *hypo-* means *below, deficient.* *(32)*

2. The prefix *para-* means *beside, near* while the prefix *peri-* means *around, about.* *(33)*

3. The prefix *inter-* means *between* while the prefix *intra-* means *within, inside.* *(32)*

4. The prefix *anti-* means *against* while the prefix *ante-* means *before.* *(32)*

5. Match the prefixes with their meanings.

_d_ endo-   (32)   _c_ a-   (32)

_a_ hemi-   (33)   _e_ post-   (33)

_f_ neo-   (32)   _b_ supra-   (32)

Part Two:

1. The suffix *-ostomy* means <u>creation of an opening</u> while the suffix *-otomy* means <u>incision into an organ</u>.   (28-29)

2. The suffix *-ectomy* means <u>surgical removal</u> while the suffix *-oscopy* means <u>visual examination</u>.   (28)

3. The suffix *-cide* means <u>kill</u> while the suffix *-cise* means <u>cut</u>.   (27-28)

4. Name three suffixes that mean *pertaining to* are <u>-ac, -al, -ic, -eal, -ary, -ous</u>.   (26)

Part Three: Match the roots with their meanings.   (30-31)

_n_ cardio   _g_ gastro   _e_ lipo
_f_ chole   _m_ gyne   _i_ litho
_a_ cranio   _d_ hepat   _h_ rhino
_l_ cysto   _k_ herni   _j_ arthro
_b_ derma   _c_ hyster

Part Four:

1. ORIF	*Open reduction internal fixation*	(35)
2. BSO	*Bilateral salpingo-oopherectomy*	(34)
3. BKA	*Below knee amputation*	(34)
4. CABG	*Coronary artery bypass graft*	(34)
5. THA	*Total hip arthroplasty*	(36)
6. TAH	*Total abdominal hysterectomy*	(36)
7. CR	*Closed reduction*	(34)

Part Five:

1. Cholecystectomy	*Removal of the gallbladder*	(38)
2. Hysterectomy	*Removal of the uterus*	(38)
3. Prostatectomy	*Removal of the prostate*	(38)

Part Six:

1. A surgical procedure to examine the thoracic cavity is called a *thoracoscopy* while the procedure to remove a lung is called a *pneumonectomy*. *(28)*

2. The surgical procedure to visually examine a joint is called an *arthroscopy* while the procedure to visually examine organs of the abdomen is called a *laparoscopy*. *(28)*

3. A colostomy is a procedure to *create a new opening to the colon* while a colectomy is a procedure to *remove a part of the large intestine (colon)*. *(28 & 31)*

4. A hysteroscopy is a *visual exam of the uterus* while a hysterectomy is a procedure to *remove the uterus*. *(28 & 31)*

Chapter 3: Anatomy for Central Service Technicians Practice Exercises

Part One:

Description	Procedure	Body System	*Page Reference*
1. Making an opening into the thoracic cavity to give surgeons access to the lungs and heart.	*Thoracotomy*	*Respiratory system*	*59*
2. Removing a salivary gland because of a tumor formation.	*Parotidectomy*	*Digestive system*	*61*
3. Removing plaque from the carotid artery that causes lack of brain oxygen.	*Carotid endarterectomy*	*Circulatory system*	*66*
4. Removing a vein from the lower limb to bypass a blocked coronary artery of the heart.	*Coronary artery bypass graft*	*Circulatory system*	*65*
5. Removal of a kidney.	*Nephrectomy*	*Urinary system*	*58*
6. Making an incision into the tympanic membrane (ear drum) to permit fluid to drain and placing small tubes in the membrane to permit continuous drainage.	*Myringotomy*	*Nervous system*	*53*
7. A repair to the muscles and ligaments of the shoulder joint.	*Rotator cuff repair*	*Muscular system*	*48*
8. Removing disc tissue pressing on the lower spine area, inserting a piece of bone between the vertebras and fusing the area with plates and screws.	*Posterior lumbar interbody fusion*	*Skeletal system*	*45*

9. Removing lymph tissue in the pharynx (throat).	*Tonsillectomy*	*Circulatory system*		65
10. Removing the gall bladder.	*Cholecystectomy*	*Digestive system*		62
11. Straightening or removing cartilage and/or bone in the nose when the nasal septum is deformed, injured or fractured.	*Septoplasty*	*Respiratory system*		60
12. Removing both fallopian tubes and ovaries.	*Bilateral salpingo-oopherectomy*	*Reproductive system*		56
13. Removing tissue or displaced bone in the wrist area to release pressure on the median nerve.	*Carpal tunnel repair*	*Nervous system*		52
14. Moving an undescended testicle.	*Orchiopexy*	*Reproductive system*		56
15. Reconstructing the ear drum so sound waves can be sent to the middle and inner ear.	*Tympanoplasty*	*Nervous system*		53

Part Two:

<u>i</u>   1.   This organ pumps blood throughout the body.   *(64)*

<u>w</u>   2.   The process by which cartilage is replaced by bone.   *(44)*

<u>j</u>   3.   Any place where two bones meet.   *(44)*

<u>k</u>   4.   The main control unit of the central nervous system.   *(49)*

<u>e</u>   5.   Considered the master gland because it helps control the activities of all other endocrine glands.   *(54)*

<u>c</u>   6.   This organ filters blood to remove amino acids and neutralize some harmful toxins.   *(58)*

<u>f</u>   7.   Produces a fluid element in semen that stimulates the motility of sperm.   *(55)*

<u>t</u>   8.   The largest part of the brain; controls mental activities and movement.   *(49)*

<u>s</u>   9.   These carry blood away from the heart.   *(64)*

<u>y</u>   10.   A somewhat flexible muscular tube that helps move food into the stomach.   *(60)*

<u>h</u>   11.   A type of connective tissue fluid that moves throughout the circulatory system.   *(63)*

<u>v</u>   12.   The pathway that food takes through the digestive system.   *(60)*

<u>b</u>   13.   Female reproductive organs.   *(55)*

<u>n</u>   14.   A cord of fibrous tissue that connects a muscle to a bone.   *(44)*

<u>m</u>   15.   The largest organ of the body.   *(43)*

_o_	16.	The basic unit of life.	(42)
_p_	17.	Tube-like structures that connect the kidneys to the urinary bladder.	(57)
_r_	18.	This is where the digestive process begins.	(60)
_u_	19.	Clear jelly-like substance that surrounds the nucleus of a cell.	(42)
_d_	20.	This part of the nervous system controls many automatic body functions like the heartbeat and breathing.	(50)

Chapter 4: Microbiology for Central Service Technicians Practice Exercises _page reference_

1. The controlling unit of a cell that governs activity and heredity is called the _nucleus._ (71)

2. Pseudomonas is sometimes called the _water bug_ because it is frequently found in water. (78)

3. _Mesophile bacteria_ are often pathogenic to humans because they grow best at body temperature. (76)

4. Herpes simplex is a _viral_ disease. (78)

5. Bacteria that require free oxygen to grow are called _aerobic_ bacteria. (75)

6. Bacteria are divided into three main shape classifications: _cocci_ (round), _bacillus_ (rods) and _spiral_ (spirals). (72)

7. Microorganisms that are capable of forming a thick wall around them to survive in adverse conditions are called _spores._ (73)

8. The two most common processes designed to classify bacteria by color change are the _gram stain_ and the _acid fast (Ziehl-Neilson stain)._ (73 & 75)

9. Tetanus and botulism do not require free oxygen to grow, so they are classified as _anaerobic_ bacteria. (75)

10. Using gram-stain classifications, _Staphylococcus_, _Enterococcus_ and _Streptococcus_ are examples of gram- _positive_ bacteria. (74)

11. The bacterial reproductive process that takes place when a mother cell divides into two daughter cells is called _binary fission_. (76)

12. Creutzfeldt-Jakob disease is caused by _prions_ which are believed to be _an abnormal form of protein_. (81)

13. _Contaminated_ is defined as the state of being soiled or infected by contact with infectious organisms or other material. (71)

14. Most bacteria are approximately _one to two_ microns in size. (72)

15. Sunlight is lethal to the _vegetative_ stage of pathogens. (76)

Chapter 5: Regulations and Standards Practice Exercises   _page reference_

| _h_ | 1. | This organization specializes in endoscopy issues and has established standards for the effective processing of flexible endoscopes. _V_ (98) |

_f_	2.	Furthers international cooperation in improving health conditions.	_V_	_(98)_
_l_	3.	Develops nationally recognized guidelines for the perioperative setting.	_V_	_(96)_
_g_	4.	Protects workers from occupationally-caused illnesses and injuries.	_R_	_(92)_
_n_	5.	Proposed standards are submitted from members such as the Association for the Advancement of Medical Instrumentation.	_V_	_(96)_
_k_	6.	Provides standards and evaluations for healthcare facilities. These evaluations are in the form of onsite surveys at least every three years.	_V_	_(97)_
_m_	7.	Creates and revises standards for processing water for irrigation.	_V_	_(97)_
_j_	8.	Creates and enforces laws relating to cleaner water, air and land.	_R_	_(92)_
_d_	9.	A voluntary international organization dedicated to the prevention and control of infections and related outcomes.	_V_	_(96)_
_e_	10.	Enforces laws relating to the transportation of medical waste.	_R_	_(91)_
_i_	11.	Is considered one of the major resources for healthcare guidelines.	_V_	_(95)_
_o_	12.	International standards to reduce the burden of fire and other hazards.	_V_	_(97)_
_a_	13.	Promotes health by preventing and controlling disease.	_V_	_(90)_
_c_	14.	Responsible for pre- and post-market medical device requirements, MedWatch, medical device classification and medical device recall.	_R_	_(87)_
_n_	15.	Enhances the global competitiveness and quality of life by promoting standards and ensuring their integrity.	_V_	_(96)_
_g & j_	16.	Agencies responsible for regulating ethylene oxide.	_R_	_(93 & 92)_
_c_	17.	Agency responsible for the MedWatch program.	_R_	_(88)_

Chapter 6: Infection Prevention and Control Practice Exercises   _page reference_

Part One: _(107-108)_

1. Decontamination: *Scrub attire; decontamination gloves; fluid resistant covering with sleeves; face mask; goggles or face shield; shoe covers*

2. Packaging area/processing area: *Scrub attire; head cover; mustache/beard cover*

3. Sterile goods storage area: *Scrub attire; head cover; mustache/beard cover*

Part Two:

1. Central Service technicians change from their street clothes into clean attire before entering their work area.

   Central Service Technicians work in a controlled environment. They help maintain that environment by removing street clothes that may carry contaminants and changing into facility issued scrubs. They wear hair covers and follow specific dress codes to reduce the amount of microorganism introduced into the work area.   *(106)*

2. Before beginning work, Central Service technicians remove jewelry.

    Watches and other jewelry can harbor microorganisms that could be transmitted into or out of the Central Service work areas.   *(106)*

3. Central Service technicians wear personal protective equipment in the decontamination area.

    Personal protective equipment is designed to protect workers in biohazard areas from bloodborne pathogen exposures that may occur as they handle contaminated items.   *(107)*

4. Food and beverages are not allowed in Central Service work areas.

    Central Service Technicians should not eat or drink in their work area for several reasons:
    *   *Beverages may spill and contaminate items.*
    *   *Food and beverages may attract insects.*
    *   *Food may cause the hands to become soiled and they may transmit bacteria.*
    *   *If hands become soiled with oils from foods, they may transmit those oils onto instruments that are going to be sterilized.*   *(113)*

5. Floors in the Central Service department should be wet mopped daily; they should never be swept or dust mopped.

    Floors in the Central Service work areas should never be swept or dust mopped because those processes cause dust to rise and it may re-deposit on items in the area. Floors in the Central Service works areas should be wet mopped at least daily.   *(114)*

Part Three: *(text page 115)*

1. *Causative agent*
2. *Reservoir of the agent*
3. *Portal of exit*
4. *Mode of transmission*
5. *Portal of entry*
6. *Susceptible host*

Chapter 7: Decontamination: Point-of-Use Preparation and Transport Practice Exercises   ***page reference***

1. The <u>*Surgery*</u> department is the major source of soiled items received by the Central Service department.   *(120)*

2. Containers dedicated to the transport of small quantities of soiled instruments should be clearly marked with a <u>*biohazard*</u> label.   *(124)*

3. When instruments are prepared for transport to the decontamination area it is important to keep them <u>*moist*</u>.   *(123)*

4. Tissue, body fat, blood and other bodily substances are examples of _gross soil_.   _(120)_

5. Disposable sharp items should be removed at the point of use and placed in a _hard-sided_ container labeled _biohazard_.   _(123)_

6. Point-of-use preparation of soiled items begins at the _decontamination_ process.   _(121)_

7. Disposable items and linen should be removed at _point of use_.   _(123)_

8. Soiled instruments should be transported in a _closed_ container or cart.   _(124)_

9. Reusable sharps should be _separated_ from other instruments and placed in a separate container so they can be _identified_ easily.   _(122)_

10. Containers and carts used to transport contaminated items should NOT be used to transport clean items unless they have been thoroughly _decontaminated_ between uses.   _(125)_

Chapter 8: Cleaning and Decontamination Practice Exercises   _page reference_

1. Instruments with lumens should always be soaked in a vertical position and should not be soaked in a horizontal position.
   b. _False_   _(153)_

2. The mechanical process by which an ultrasonic cleaner works is called cavitation.
   a. _True_   _(139)_

3. To prevent aerosols, items should be brushed below the surface of the water.
   a. _True_   _(153)_

4. Automatic washers clean using a spray-force action called impingement.
   a. _True_   _(141)_

5. Instruments received from surgery and tagged for repair do not need to be cleaned until they come back from repair.
   b. _False_   _(154)_

6. Powered surgical instruments should be cleaned using a mechanical cleaning process.
   b. _False_   _(157)_

7. There are currently no methods available to verify cleaning process outcomes.
   b. _False_   _(158)_

8. All sonic cleaners have a decontamination cycle.
   b. _False_   _(139)_

9. Horizontal work surfaces in the decontamination area should be cleaned and disinfected once per day.
   b. _False_   _(133)_

10. Because of the cavitation and impingement action of mechanical cleaners, there is no need to pre-clean items that will be processed in a mechanical cleaner.
   b. _False_   _(139)_

Chapter 9: Disinfection Practice Exercises   <u>*page reference*</u>

Part One:

<u>d</u> 1. The use of heat to kill all microorganisms except spores.   *(173)*

<u>b</u> 2. A chemical which kills most pathogenic organisms, but does not kill spores. *(163)*

<u>a</u> 3. A solution which inhibits the growth of bacteria usually used topically
        and only on animate objects.   *(165)*

<u>h</u> 4. The length of time an item must remain wet with a disinfectant.   *(173)*

<u>j</u> 5. The destruction of nearly all pathogenic microorganisms on an inanimate
        surface.   *(163)*

<u>c</u> 6. Relating to the destruction of bacteria.   *(163)*

<u>k</u> 7. The frequency the concentration level of a high-level disinfectant must
        be tested.   *(175)*

<u>e</u> 8. A process by which all forms of microbial life are destroyed.   *(163)*

<u>f</u> 9. Minimum effective concentration testing is required when using this
        disinfectant.   *(169)*

<u>m</u> 10. When manually disinfecting lumens, care should be taken to ensure
        there are no _____present inside the lumens.   *(173)*

Part Two:

1. This low-level disinfectant is often used in environmental sanitation such as on floors, walls and furniture. It is incompatible with soaps. Its concentration may be diminished by some materials such as cotton, wool, filter paper and charcoal.

    It is: <u>*Quaternary Ammonium compounds*</u>   *(164)*

2. This high-level disinfectant is used for semi-critical devices such as endoscopes. Once it is activated (mixed) it must be checked routinely using test strips to ensure its concentration. Because of its fumes employees who work with it must follow specific Occupational Safety and Health Administration guidelines for safety.

    It is: <u>*Glutaraldehyde*</u>   *(167)*

3. This common disinfectant has been in use for several years. It is often used to disinfect equipment. It is inactivated by organic soil. In order to achieve a reasonable level of disinfection, it must remain in wet contact with the item being disinfected for at least five minutes; this can be a problem because it evaporates quickly.

    It is: <u>*Alcohol*</u>   *(165)*

4. This intermediate-level disinfectant is a member of the halogen disinfectant family. Although it may be found in Central Service decontamination areas, it is not recommended for use on instruments because of its corrosive qualities.

    It is: <u>*Chlorine*</u>   *(167)*

Part One:

<u>*l*</u>   1.   A self-retaining retractor.   *(188)*

<u>*e*</u>   2.   The part of a ring-handled surgical instrument that locks the handles in place. *(183)*

<u>*b*</u>   3.   Surgical instruments used to cut away at bone and tissue.   *(182)*

<u>*d*</u>   4.   A chemical process applied during instrument manufacture that provides a
              corrosion-resistant finish.   *(183)*

<u>*c*</u>   5.   Also known as 400 series stainless steel, this metal used in surgical instrument
              manufacturing can be heat hardened.   *(181)*

<u>*h*</u>   6.   Surgical instruments used to cut, incise or dissect tissue.   *(182)*

<u>*f*</u>   7.   Commonly found in the Operating Room, this can damage instruments with
              prolonged exposure.   *(194)*

<u>*g*</u>   8.   Surgical instruments used to grasp.   *(182)*

<u>*k*</u>   9.   Where the two parts of a ring-handled instrument meet and pivot.   *(183)*

<u>*o*</u>   10.   Inserts for needle holders are frequently made of this metal.   *(186)*

Part Two:

1. Tungsten carbide scissors blades hold a sharp edge longer than stainless steel blades.
    a. *True*   *(190)*

2. Tissue forceps have teeth and dressing forceps have serrations.
    a. *True*   *(186-87)*

3. Double-action rongeurs should be tested for sharpness using tissue paper.
    b. *False*   *(197)*

4. Laser etching is an acceptable method for marking instruments.
    a. *True*   *(199)*

5. Because they are mild cleaners, dish soaps are the cleaners of choice for surgical
    instruments.
    b. *False*   *(195)*

Part Three: *(184)*

    a. *Tip*
    b. *Jaw*
    c. *Box lock*
    d. *Shank*
    e. *Ratchet*
    f. *Ring handle*

Chapter 11: Complex Surgical Instruments Practice Exercises *page reference*

Part One: *(209)*

_d_ 1. Used to repair and reconstruct teeth and jawbones.

_e_ 2. Used in ear surgery and for driving very small wires through bone.

_c_ 3. Used in open heart surgery.

_b_ 4. Used to remove cement.

_a_ 5. Used to harvest skin grafts and reshape skin surfaces.

_f_ 6. Used to perform specific cutting actions such as reciprocating or oscillating.

Part Two: *(221-22)*

_d_ 1. Allows for visual inspection of the lower part of the large intestine.

_c_ 2. Allows for visual inspection of the upper digestive tract.

_b_ 3. Used to visualize the urethra and bladder.

_a_ 4. Used to visualize the tracheobronchial tree.

_e_ 5. Used to visualize the entire large intestine.

Part Three:

1. Leak testing should be performed on each flexible endoscope on an annual basis.
    b. *False* *(223)*

2. Loaner instrument trays that are received sterile from other facilities do not need to be decontaminated and re-sterilized before use.
    b. *False* *(240)*

3. Endoscope channels should be cleaned and then left moist for storage.
    b. *False* *(232)*

4. Powered surgical instruments have one of three power sources: electricity, air or battery.
    a. *True* *(205)*

5. Modern powered surgical instruments can be immersed.
    b. *False* *(205)*

6. Laparoscopic instrument insulation failure can cause burns.
    a. *True* *(217)*

7. The purpose of a decontamination battery is to protect powered surgical instruments from fluid invasion.
    a. *True* *(210)*

8. Dental drills are used to remove cement.
    b. *False* *(209)*

9. Automatic endoscope reprocessors are not recommended for flexible endoscopes.
    b. *False* *(227)*

Chapter 12: Assembly and Packaging Practice Exercises *page reference*

_j_   1.   An acceptable method of package closure that is also used as an external indicator.   *(283)*

_h_   2.   Minimum amount of time that packaging materials should be held at room temperature and at 30% to 70% relative humidity before sterilization.   *(287)*

_l_   3.   Flat wrapping technique that applies one wrap on top of another to create a package within a package.   *(271)*

_c_   4.   Government agency that regulates sterilization packaging materials.   *(259)*

_p_   5.   This type of packaging contains no cellulosic materials and would be used to package small items for low-temperature sterilization.   *(266)*

_i_   6.   This type of packaging can be used in steam and ethylene oxide sterilization but is not recommended for other types of sterilization.   *(266)*

_b_   7.   When using paper/plastic pouches, package content information should be written on this side of the pouch.   *(286)*

_k_   8.   This is NOT an acceptable method of package closure.   *(285)*

_e_   9.   Muslin is an example of this type of packaging material.   *(260)*

_o_   10.   The wrapping technique most commonly used for small packs and most trays.   *(270)*

Chapter 13: Point-of-Use Processing Practice Exercises *page reference*

1. Sterilization documentation is not required for items that are steam sterilized for immediate use.
   - b. *False*   *(297)*

2. Instruments must be cleaned before being sterilized for immediate use.
   - a. *True*   *(295)*

3. Personal protective equipment is not required when cleaning items for Immediate Use Steam Sterilization.
   - b. *False*   *(295)*

4. The sterilization method of choice for single-use items is Immediate Use Steam Sterilization.
   - b. *False*   *(295)*

5. It is recommended to use Immediate Use Steam Sterilization to sterilize instruments contaminated with Creutzfeldt-Jakob disease after the procedure has been completed.
   - b. *False*   *(295)*

6. Immediate Use Steam Sterilization was developed to process items when the facility does not have enough instruments to perform the surgery.
   - b. *False*   *(292)*

7. To sterilize items using steam, the item's manufacturer instructions must state the item can be sterilized using an immediate use steam sterilization cycle.
   a. True   *(293)*

8. When processing items for immediate use, items do not need to be disassembled prior to cleaning.
   b. False   *(295)*

9. When using low-temperature methods for sterilization or disinfection of items at the point of use, item preparation is not as critical as when preparing items for terminal sterilization.
   b. False   *(298)*

10. All items sterilized or high-level disinfected at the point of use must be carefully monitored and logged.
   a. True   *(298)*

Chapter 14: High-Temperature Sterilization Practice Exercises   *page reference*

1. The interior chamber walls of the sterilizer are heated by steam in the *jacket* of the sterilizer.   *(304)*

2. The *gasket* is designed to maintain a tight seal that prevents steam from escaping the chamber of a sterilizer.   *(305)*

3. The *chamber drain* is located in the floor of the steam sterilizer.   *(305)*

4. The portion of the steam sterilizer that measures steam temperature and automatically controls the flow of air and condensate from the sterilizer chamber is the *thermomatic strip*.   *(306)*

5. *Charts and printouts* provide a written record of sterilizer cycle activities.   *(306)*

6. *Gravity* sterilizers remove air from the chamber by steam forcing the cooler air in the chamber out through the drain.   *(307)*

7. The most frequent cause for sterilization failure is lack of steam *contact*.   *(311)*

8. Inadequate *exposure* time at the correct elevated temperature is a reason for sterilization failure.   *(312)*

9. Another name for superheated steam is *dry* steam.   *(313)*

10. Placing warm sterilized packages on cool surfaces will cause *condensate* to form. *(317)*

Chapter 15: Low-Temperature Sterilization Practice Exercises   *page reference*

1. *Oxygen* is a byproduct of ozone sterilization.   *(335)*

2. The *ethylene oxide* method of low-temperature sterilization uses gas cartridges for a sterilant.   *(324)*

3. The probability of a viable microorganism being present on an item after sterilization is the *sterility assurance level.*   *(322)*

4. The bacterial spore used to test ethylene oxide sterilization cycles is _Bacillus atrophaeus_. *(327)*

5. Cycle time for items sterilized using ozone sterilization is _4.5 hours_. *(335)*

6. An aeration time of _eight hours_ at 140⁰ F is recommended for items sterilized with ethylene oxide. *(327)*

7. _Geobacillus stearothermophilus_ is a bacterial spore used to test hydrogen peroxide sterilization cycles. *(332 & 335)*

8. Exposure time for items sterilized using ethylene oxide sterilization is _2.5 hours_. *(325)*

9. _The Occupational Safety and Health Administration_ sets exposure standards for chemical sterilants. *(323)*

10. _U.S. Food and Drug Administration_ recommends that sterilants be rigorously tested before being marketed. *(322)*

Chapter 16: Sterile Storage and Transport Practice Exercises   *page reference*

_p_   1.   _____is a method of stock rotation which ensures that older items are used first. *(352)*

_a_   2.   Air flow in the sterile storage area should be _____. *(344)*

_l_   3.   Packaging that prevents microorganisms from entering the packages and allows aseptic opening is called_____. *(342)*

_n_   4.   Humidity in the sterile storage area should be _____. *(344)*

_b_   5.   Temperature in the sterile storage area should be_____. *(344)*

_o_   6.   The _____ shelf of storage carts should be solid. *(346)*

_j_   7.   Items _____ be used after the manufacturer's expiration date as long as the package integrity is still intact. *(349)*

_c_   8.   Stacking rigid containers too high can cause _____ damage. *(347)*

_k_   9.   Items should be stored at least ____ inches below sprinkler heads. *(350)*

_i_   10.   When transporting sterile items in a dedicated clean lift they _____ be contained. *(354)*

Chapter 17: Monitoring and Recordkeeping for Central Service Practice Exercises

_m_   1.   The _____ is the dating system that uses the number of days that have elapsed in the year. *(366)*

_a_   2.   Keeping records accurate and complete is important because they are used during The Joint Commission and Centers for Medicare and Medicaid Services surveys, but may also be used in _____. *(358)*

_b_ 3. _____records are kept to provide evidence that an employee has kept current and is aware of new best practices. *(371)*

_r_ 4. A _____ should be run in every sterilizer load that contains implants. *(365)*

_d_ 5. Recording _____ is an example of formal monitoring. *(359)*

_c_ 6. Label that contains the date, sterilizer identification and sterilizer cycle number is called a _____. *(366)*

_p_ 7. _____are used to help determine where employees excel or where they may need additional training. *(371)*

_e_ 8. Ultrasonic cleaners clean by a process called _____. *(360)*

_i_ 9. A test performed to help ensure there are no air leaks in a steam sterilizer is called a _____. *(368)*

_g_ 10. If there is no bacterial growth in a biological indicator after sterilization and incubation it is called a _____ test. *(364)*

Chapter 18: Quality Assurance Practice Exercises *page reference*

1. Nurses, physicians and other professionals working in a healthcare facility are *internal* customers of Central Service. *(374)*

2. An activity designed to identify and resolve work task-related problems is called *process improvement*. *(376)*

3. The consistent delivery of products and services according to established standards is called *quality*. *(374)*

4. The *patient* must be the center of every quality concern. *(374)*

5. A process that looks backwards at an event to help prevent it from reoccurring is called a *root cause analysis*. *(380)*

6. The quality process that uses DMADV/DMAIC to improve processes is called *Six Sigma*. *(383)*

7. *ISO 9000* is an international standard used by participating organizations to help assure that they consistently deliver quality services and products. *(386)*

8. The act of granting authority to employees to make decisions within their areas of responsibility is called *empowerment*. *(376)*

9. A series of work activities which produce a product or service is called a *work process*. *(381)*

10. An unexpected occurrence involving death, serious physical or psychological injury or the risk thereof is called a *sentinel event*. *(381)*

Chapter 19: Managing Inventory within the Central Service Department Practice Exercises *page reference*

Part One:

1. When items are needed immediately (at once) Central Service technicians may receive a *STAT* order. *(403)*

2. Something of value that is owned by an organization or person is called an _asset_. *(394)*

3. Detergents, sterilization quality assurance products and other items that are purchased, used up and replaced are called _consumable inventory_. *(394)*

4. Sterilizers, mechanical washers and other expensive items are examples of _capital_ equipment. *(394)*

5. The act of moving supplies throughout the facility is called _distribution_. *(396)*

6. Process designed to reduce harm to the environment is called _sustainability_. *(402)*

Part Two:

1. Name the system: _Exchange cart_ *(400)*

2. Name the system: _Case cart_ *(401)*

3. Name the system: _Requisition_ *(401)*

4. Name the system: _Periodic automated replenishment_ *(399)*

5. Name the system: _Automated supply replenishment system_ *(399)*

Part Three: *(396)*

1. _Do not reuse (single use)_

2. _Lot number_

3. _Manufacture date_

4. _Reference (catalog) number_

5. _Serial number_

6. _Expiration date_

Chapter 20: The Role of Central Service in Ancillary Department Support Practice Exercises

Part One: __page reference__

_g_ 1. The department that checks patient care equipment for safety and function. *(410)*

_f_ 2. Allows the patient to self-administer pain medication. *(409)*

<u>a</u> 3. Applies a brief electroshock to restore the rhythm of the heart. *(409)*

<u>b</u> 4. Artificially stimulates the venous plantar plexus to increase circulation in bed-ridden patients. *(409)*

<u>l</u> 5. This device moves joints after surgery or trauma. *(409)*

<u>e</u> 6. This unit is used to raise or lower body temperature. *(409)*

Part Two: <u>*page reference*</u>

1. Manufacturers sometimes loan equipment to facilities at no cost if the facility agrees to purchase disposable equipment components from the manufacturer.
    a. *True* *(414)*

2. A gastric suction unit is used to suction liquids from oral and nasal cavities.
    b. *False* *(409)*

3. Both Biomedical technicians and Central Service technicians are qualified to repair patient care equipment.
    b. *False* *(410)*

4. Used equipment that is not visibly soiled may be returned to the clean equipment storage area without undergoing a decontamination process.
    b. *False* *(410)*

Chapter 21: The Role of Information Technology in Central Service Practice Exercises

1. List six reasons why it is important for the Central Service department to track items. *(418)*

    1. *Ensure items can be quickly located*
    2. *Determine when consumable supplies should be replaced*
    3. *Monitor item usage*
    4. *Maintain accurate records of processes*
    5. *Assist with quality assurance processes and regulatory compliance*
    6. *Capture information for financial analysis*

2. Interfaced, cloud based or turnkey: which of these terms means systems communicate with each other? *Interfaced.* *(419)*

3. Name two types of tracking systems.

    Standard bar codes
    Radio frequency identification tags *(423)*

4. List three things a basic instrument and equipment tracking system can track. *(425-26)*
    1. *Instruments and trays*
    2. *Specific equipment items*
    3. *Last known location of a specific instrument set*
    4. *Cost and value of specific equipment and instruments*
    5. *Number of complete processing and use cycles*
    6. *Usage of specific equipment*
    7. *Preventive maintenance schedules*

Chapter 22: Safety and Risk Management for Central Service Practice Exercises

Part One: *page reference*

1. The three types of hazards found in the Central Service department are *physical*,
    biological and *chemical*.   *(431)*

2. The methods used to assess the risks of a specific activity, and to develop a program to
    reduce losses from exposure to those risks is called *risk management.*   *(430)*

3. You would find physical data relating to a chemical on the *safety data sheet.* *(436)*

4. Occupational Safety and Health Administration has established permissible exposure
    limits for many chemicals like hydrogen peroxide and ozone as *one ppm.* *(437)*

5. The three elements that make up the fire triangle are *combustible substance,*
    source of oxygen and *source of ignition.*   *(438)*

Part Two:

1. If an injury seems insignificant, there is no need to report it.
    b. *False*   *(448)*

2. Preparation and sterilization areas pose no risk of injury to Central Service technicians.
    b. *False*   *(441)*

3. Gas cylinder regulators are interchangeable between different types of gases.
    b. *False*   *(446)*

4. Loss of the Central Service department's water supply would be an example of an
    internal disaster.
    a. *True*   *(447)*

5. Part of a facilities employee training plan should include emergency spill procedures
    and how to read safety data sheets.
    a. *True*   *(449)*

Part Three:

___	Asbestos		_x_	Needle sticks and punctures *(434)*
_x_	Ethylene oxide *(442)*		___	Freons
___	Radiation		___	Paints and solvents
___	Mercury		_x_	Bloodborne pathogens *(431)*
_x_	Infectious agents *(431)*		_x_	Ergonomic stressors *(432)*
___	Boiler compounds		_x_	Burns *(433)*
_x_	Chemicals *(431)*		_x_	Falls *(433)*
___	Adhesives		___	Chemical fixers and developer

Chapter 23: Success through Communication Practice Exercises   *page reference*

_j_   1.   The sequence of steps used to address customer complaints.   *(464)*

_g_   2.   Positive reinforcement used to encourage employees to
           follow proper work practices and negative reinforcement
           to discourage inappropriate work practices.   *(457)*

_f_   3.   This communication process occurs when the listener asks a question, repeats information or otherwise helps the speaker to know if the message has been correctly received. *(455)*

_c_   4.   Behavior relating to what is right or wrong relative to the standards of conduct for a profession. *(455)*

_a_   5.   The process of transmitting information and understanding from one person to another by use of words and non-verbal expressions such as body language. *(455)*

_i_   6.   The broad range of human characteristics and dimensions which impact an employee's values, opportunities and perceptions of themselves and others at work. *(463)*

Chapter 24: Personal and Professional Development for Central Service Practice Exercises

<u>*page reference*</u>

_e_   1.   Developing professional resources in the field of Central Service can provide a _____ to share information. *(471)*

_i_   2.   Attending educational _____ is one way to help achieve career goals. *(471)*

_b_   3.   One of the most important factors in attaining goals is finding the right _____. *(471)*

_c_   4.   _____ identifies and develops talent as well as improves employability. *(468)*

_h_   5.   "Do you like your job?" is an example of a/an _____ question. *(473)*

_j_   6.   A _____ is a compilation of skills, education and accomplishments. *(471)*

REVIEW QUIZZES

Chapter 1: Introduction to Central Service Review Quiz

Complete the following 10 multiple choice questions.

1. Soiled instruments and other items are received in the _____ area of the Central Service department.
   a. preparation
   b. packaging
   c. decontamination
   d. sterilization

2. The first step in the sterilization process is
   a. receiving.
   b. sorting.
   c. soaking.
   d. cleaning.

3. Central Service technicians must wear special attire referred to as _____ to minimize their exposure to bloodborne pathogens and other contaminants.
   a. PPE
   b. OSHA
   c. TPA
   d. CDC

4. Instrument sets and other required instrumentation needed for all scheduled procedures for an entire day are usually pulled (collected)
   a. two days before they will be used.
   b. the day or evening before they will be used.
   c. the morning of the planned surgery.
   d. early morning (for morning procedures) and early afternoon (for afternoon procedures) on the day of surgery.

5. The use of analytical skills to solve problems and make decisions is a component of which of the following knowledge and skills dimensions?
   a. Communication abilities
   b. Facility system responsibilities
   c. Employability skills
   d. Safety practices

6. Healthcare-associated infections are
   a. most likely to occur during a surgical procedure.
   b. caused by drug resistant organisms.
   c. infections without known cures.
   d. infections which occur in the course of being treated in a healthcare facility.

7. The human resources tool that defines job duties performed by persons in specific positions is called a
    a. job duty list.
    b. job specification.
    c. task summary review.
    d. job description.

8. In the future, which of the following will more frequently become a requirement for working in a Central Service department?
    a. On-the-job training
    b. Experience
    c. Formal education
    d. Reference from facility administrator

9. While items may be dispensed to all areas of a facility, the major focus of the sterile storage personnel is
    a. the Emergency Department.
    b. Labor & Delivery.
    c. Materiel Management.
    d. the Operating Room.

10. Which of the following is NOT a growing trend in Central Service?
    a. Decentralization of Central Service responsibilities
    b. The use of more reusable and more complex devices
    c. Satellite-processing units with centralized management
    d. Consolidation into entire integrated delivery networks

Chapter 2: Medical Terminology for Central Service Technicians
Review Quiz

Complete the following 20 multiple choice questions.

1. Knowing and understanding medical terminology helps technicians
   a. reduce the productivity of the Operating Room.
   b. understand manufacturer's Instructions for Use.
   c. understand what is asked when a request is made.
   d. become proficient in Latin and French word elements.

2. The majority of medical terms are of either _____ or _____ origin.
   a. Greek or French
   b. Greek or Latin
   c. Latin or French
   d. Latin or English

3. Which of the following tells the primary meaning of a word?
   a. Prefix word element
   b. Root word element
   c. Suffix word element
   d. Combining vowel

4. The purpose of a combining vowel is to
   a. tell the primary meaning of a word.
   b. suggest the meaning of the root word element.
   c. ease pronunciation of a word.
   d. connect the prefix and the suffix.

5. The last word element in a medical term is the
   a. combining vowel.
   b. prefix.
   c. suffix.
   d. root.

6. The term *itis* means
   a. illness.
   b. inflammation.
   c. the study of.
   d. pain.

7. The term *ectomy* means
   a. to repair.
   b. surgical removal.
   c. inflammation.
   d. to cut.

8. The term *oscopy* means
   a. visual examination.
   b. disease.
   c. surgical removal.
   d. diagnosis of a medical condition.

9. Arthroscopy means
   a. visual exam of a joint.
   b. surgical replacement of a joint.
   c. inflammation of a joint.
   d. surgical removal of a joint.

10. The term *ostomy*
   a. is a prefix.
   b. is a suffix.
   c. is a root.
   d. means surgical removal.

11. The suffix *-tome* means a
   a. surgical restoration.
   b. surgical fixation.
   c. to suture.
   d. cutting instrument.

12. *Plasty* is a
   a. prefix meaning to suture.
   b. prefix meaning surgical restoration.
   c. suffix meaning surgical restoration.
   d. is a suffix meaning to view.

13. The word *laminectomy* means
   a. removal of a cyst in the spine.
   b. removal of part of a lamina.
   c. to cut out part of a small bone.
   d. the study of the spine.

14. Which of the following means *beside* or *near*?
   a. Para
   b. Peri
   c. Parta
   d. Pana

15. Which of the following surgical abbreviations might be used relating to a fractured bone?
   a. CABG
   b. BSO
   c. ORIF
   d. TAH

16. The term *intercostal* means
     a.   within the colon.
     b.   between the toes.
     c.   within the bladder.
     d.   between the ribs.

17. The term *hypo* means
     a.   quickly.
     b.   above.
     c.   below.
     d.   measured.

18. The term *septorhinoplasty* means
     a.   surgery of a muscle wound.
     b.   surgical repair of the nose.
     c.   removal of a cyst.
     d.   incision of the stomach.

19. Encephalopathy is a/an
     a.   disease of the brain.
     b.   inflammation of the liver.
     c.   fluid-filled sack.
     d.   inflammation of a joint.

20. Lithotripsy means
     a.   aspiration of fatty tissue.
     b.   surgical removal of the ovary.
     c.   crushing of a stone.
     d.   visual examination of a joint.

Chapter 3: Anatomy for Central Service Technicians Review Quiz

Complete the following 20 multiple choice questions.

1. This system gives the body shape and support.
   a. Muscular system
   b. Nervous system
   c. Skeletal system
   d. Circulatory system

2. This tissue acts as a cushion between bones to prevent them from rubbing together.
   a. Tendon
   b. Muscle
   c. Cartilage
   d. Ligament

3. These muscles control involuntary movements like breathing, digestion, etc.
   a. Smooth
   b. Cardiac
   c. Skeletal
   d. Fascia

4. This surgical procedure consists of removing an ear bone that has thickened and no longer transmits sound waves and replacing it with an artificial implant to improve hearing.
   a. Tympanoplasty
   b. Stapedectomy
   c. Auditory implantation
   d. Myringotomy

5. More than 55% of blood is made up of this yellowish liquid.
   a. Platelets
   b. Red blood cells
   c. White blood cells
   d. Plasma

6. The organ that filters the blood to remove amino acids and neutralize some harmful toxins.
   a. Kidney
   b. Pancreas
   c. Liver
   d. Gall bladder

7. This surgical procedure removes the uterus.
   a. Hysteroscopy
   b. Hysterectomy
   c. Dilation & curettage
   d. Bilateral salpingo-oophorectomy

8. This gland stimulates body growth.
    a. Adrenal
    b. Thyroid
    c. Pancreas
    d. Pituitary

9. This is the lining of the uterus.
    a. Vagina
    b. Endometrium
    c. Fimbriae
    d. Skin

10. This surgical procedure removes tissue or displaced bone from the wrist area to release pressure on the median nerve.
    a. Carpal tunnel repair
    b. Ulnar nerve transposition
    c. Arthrotomy
    d. Fasciotomy

11. The largest part of the human brain is the
    a. brain stem.
    b. cerebellum.
    c. cerebrum.
    d. spinal cord.

12. This surgical procedure is the relocation of an undescended testicle.
    a. Transurethral resection
    b. Prostatectomy
    c. Orchiopexy
    d. Orchiectomy

13. The throat is also called the
    a. esophagus.
    b. larynx.
    c. trachea.
    d. pharynx.

14. This surgical procedure is the removal of the gall bladder.
    a. Cholecystectomy
    b. Colectomy
    c. Parotidectomy
    d. Gastrectomy

15. The hip joint is an example of a
    a. gliding joint.
    b. ball and socket joint.
    c. pivot joint.
    d. hinge joint.

16. This tissue covers the body's external surface.
     a. Epithelial tissue
     b. Connective tissue
     c. Muscular tissue
     d. Nervous tissue

17. The brain center of a cell is the
     a. cell membrane.
     b. cytoplasm.
     c. nucleus.
     d. deoxyribonucleic acid.

18. Cartilage is replaced by bone through a process called
     a. ossification.
     b. calcification.
     c. osmosis.
     d. cancellous formation.

19. The white portion of the eye is called the
     a. retina.
     b. iris.
     c. pupil.
     d. sclera.

20. This is referred to as the voice box.
     a. Pharynx
     b. Larynx
     c. Mouth
     d. Trachea

Chapter 4: Microbiology for Central Service Technicians Review Quiz

Indicate whether each of the following 10 statements is true or false.

1. Healthy people do not harbor or transmit bacteria.
   a. True
   b. False

2. Anaerobic bacteria require free oxygen to live.
   a. True
   b. False

3. Viruses are larger than bacteria.
   a. True
   b. False

4. The spore is the control unit of a cell.
   a. True
   b. False

5. Staphylococcus is classified as a gram-positive bacteria.
   a. True
   b. False

6. All microorganisms are harmful to humans.
   a. True
   b. False

7. Spores help some microorganisms survive in adverse conditions.
   a. True
   b. False

8. All bacteria require the same conditions to live and grow.
   a. True
   b. False

9. Psychrophiles grow best in warm temperatures.
   a. True
   b. False

10. When cleaning prion-contaminated instruments no special cleaning procedures are required, only following standard cleaning protocols and the manufacturer's Instructions for Use is necessary.
    a. True
    b. False

Complete the following five multiple choice questions.

11. Microorganisms reproduce by a process called
    a. repopulation.
    b. binary fission.
    c. replication.
    d. bilateral reproduction.

12. Bacteria that cause disease are called
    a. gram positive.
    b. gram negative.
    c. pathogens.
    d. potentially infectious.

13. The part of a cell that controls cell function is the
    a. cytoplasm.
    b. nucleus.
    c. cell membrane.
    d. capsule.

14. The virus that causes hepatitis B is transmitted by
    a. contact.
    b. blood.
    c. airborne.
    d. vector borne.

15. _____ is an example of a fungus.
    a. Pneumonia
    b. Tuberculosis
    c. Athlete's foot
    d. Herpes simplex

Chapter 5: Regulations and Standards Review Quiz

Complete the following 10 multiple choice questions.

1. Agency which may intervene in a matter of worker protection even if there are no specific regulations covering the situation.
   - a. Occupational Safety and Health Administration
   - b. Environmental Protection Agency
   - c. U.S. Food and Drug Administration
   - d. Association of periOperative Registered Nurses

2. Regulations under the Clean Air Act are administered by the
   - a. Occupational Safety and Health Administration.
   - b. U.S. Food and Drug Administration.
   - c. Environmental Protection Agency.
   - d. Association of periOperative Registered Nurses.

3. The agency which imposes very strict labeling requirements on manufacturers of disinfectants used by Central Service departments.
   - a. Occupational Safety and Health Administration
   - b. U.S. Food and Drug Administration
   - c. Environmental Protection Agency
   - d. Association for the Advancement of Medical Instrumentation

4. Healthcare regulations and standards establish
   - a. minimal levels of quality and safety.
   - b. equal pay practices.
   - c. productivity time lines.
   - d. all of the above.

5. Chemical indicators are classified as
   - a. FDA Class I medical devices.
   - b. FDA Class II medical devices.
   - c. FDA Class III medical devices.
   - d. none, not regulated by FDA.

6. Heart valves and pacemakers are examples of
   - a. FDA Class I medical devices.
   - b. FDA Class II medical devices.
   - c. FDA Class III medical devices.
   - d. none, not regulated by FDA.

7. Under current regulations, who is required to report suspected medical device-related deaths to the U.S. Food and Drug Administration?
   - a. Device manufacturer
   - b. Hospitals
   - c. All of the above
   - d. None of the above

8. Standards and regulations help set levels of _____ in our departments.
   a. quality
   b. safety
   c. efficiency
   (d.) both quality and safety

9. Medical device reporting is regulated by the
   a. National Fire Protection Association
   b. Environmental Protection Agency
   c. World Health Organization
   (d.) U.S. Food and Drug Administration

10. The Department of Transportation enforces statutes relating to the
    a. transportation of clean and soiled instruments between facilities.
    (b.) transportation of unclean, damaged flexible endoscopes.
    c. transportation of equipment for the decontamination area.
    d. transportation of instrumentation across state lines.

Indicate whether each of the following 10 statements is true or false.

11. Sometimes state or local regulations differ from Federal regulations and when that happens, the most stringent regulations apply.
    (a.) True
    b. False

12. Following the Occupational Safety and Health Administration's regulations for wearing personal protective equipment in the Central Service decontamination area is optional.
    a. True
    (b.) False

13. Third-party reprocessors are regulated by the U.S. Food and Drug Administration.
    (a.) True
    b. False

14. Recommendations regarding sterilization practices are provided by the Association for the Advancement of Medical Instrumentation.
    (a.) True
    b. False

15. The American National Standards Institute is a voluntary association dedicated to infection control and prevention.
    a. True
    (b.) False

16. Failure to receive accreditation from The Joint Commission can result in the loss of Medicare and Medicaid payments.
    (a.) True
    b. False

17. The Society of Gastroenterology Nurses and Associates is a source for information about the proper processing of flexible endoscopes.
    a. True
    b. False

18. Class III medical devices are identified as high risk.
    a. True
    b. False

19. Reuse of single use medical devices is less regulated now than it was in the 1990's.
    a. True
    b. False

20. The U.S. Food and Drug Administration recalls may be either mandatory or voluntary.
    a. True
    b. False

Chapter 6: Infection Prevention and Control Review Quiz

Complete the following 15 multiple choice questions.

1. Each year, approximately _____ patients develop a healthcare-associated infection.
   a. 1 million
   b. 2 million
   c. 700,000
   d. 500,000

2. Jewelry should NOT be worn in the Central Service department work areas because they
   a. harbor bacteria.
   b. are expensive.
   c. may be damaged.
   d. may be misplaced or stolen.

3. During handwashing, hands should be lathered and scrubbed for at least
   a. 10 seconds
   b. 20 seconds
   c. 1 minute
   d. 2 minutes

4. To protect themselves from splashes and spills, Central Service technicians assigned to the decontamination area should wear
   a. double-cloth gowns.
   b. blue surgical scrubs.
   c. fluid-resistant gowns.
   d. sterile Operating Room gowns.

5. The main theory of standard precautions is
   a. that patients in high-risk categories may be infectious.
   b. that patients diagnosed with a specific disease may be infectious.
   c. that patients are generally healthy unless they show symptoms of an infectious disease.
   d. to treat all human blood and bodily fluids as infectious.

6. Which of the following is NOT a requirement of the Occupational Safety and Health Administration Bloodborne Pathogen Standard?
   a. Provide hepatitis B vaccine to employees at no cost
   b. Observe standard precautions
   c. Keep biohazard areas locked
   d. Use engineering controls to prevent biohazard exposures

7. The only way to interrupt the transmission of a causative agent is to
   a. sterilize the item.
   b. wear appropriate personal protective equipment.
   c. eliminate it.
   d. involve the Occupational Safety and Health Administration.

8. Departmental dress codes applies to
   a. everyone entering the Central Service department.
   b. only hospital employees.
   c. only persons who will be spending more than 10 minutes in the Central Service work area.
   d. only visitors such as sales reps, maintenance personnel, etc.

9. Inanimate objects that can transmit bacteria are called
   a. transmission devices.
   b. fomites.
   c. carriers.
   d. framiseals.

10. Floors in the Central Service department should be
    a. wet-mopped daily.
    b. wet-mopped weekly.
    c. swept daily and wet-mopped weekly.
    d. swept daily.

11. The absence of microorganisms that cause disease is called
    a. infection prevention.
    b. infection control.
    c. asepsis.
    d. HIA control.

12. Know what is dirty, know what is clean, know what is sterile; keeping the three conditions separate and remedying contamination immediately are known as
    a. the principles of asepsis.
    b. the basics of the Bloodborne Pathogen Standard.
    c. the principles of infection prevention and control.
    d. the basics of environmental control.

13. What color should biohazard labels/signs be?
    a. Red/orange
    b. Orange/yellow
    c. Orange/blue
    d. Green/black

14. The decontamination area of the Central Service department should have
    a. negative air flow.
    b. positive air flow.
    c. filtered air flow.
    d. no air exchanges because it is a biohazard area.

15. Which of these traffic control/dress code requirements applies to the clean assembly area of Central Service?
    a. Biohazard
    b. Unrestricted
    c. Semi restricted
    d. Restricted

Chapter 7: Decontamination: Point-of-Use Preparation and Transport Review Quiz

Indicate whether each of the following 10 statements is true or false.

1. Items that have been used in patient care should be considered contaminated.
   - **a.** True
   - b. False

2. If soiled items are held in user units before pick up for processing, they must be kept at the patient's bedside until Central Service collects them.
   - a. True
   - **b.** False

3. To prevent the growth of biofilm, soil on used instruments should be allowed to dry.
   - a. True
   - **b.** False

4. Users are responsible to notify Central Service if they discover instruments or equipment that need repair.
   - **a.** True
   - b. False

5. It is acceptable to transport soiled and clean items at the same time in the same cart if they are placed on separate shelves.
   - a. True
   - **b.** False

6. When moving transport carts throughout the healthcare facility, Central Service technicians must always yield right of way to patients and visitors.
   - **a.** True
   - b. False

7. Failure to perform soiled pick-up rounds as scheduled can lead to instrument and equipment shortages.
   - **a.** True
   - b. False

8. Everyone who may transport contaminated items must be trained in safe handling.
   - **a.** True
   - b. False

9. When it is necessary to transport soiled items between facilities using a truck or van, facilities must consult the U.S. Department of Transportation, as well as state and local laws for transporting biohazardous items.
   - **a.** True
   - b. False

10. One goal of point-of-use preparation is to prevent instruments from being damaged.
    - **a.** True
    - b. False

Chapter 8: Cleaning and Decontamination Review Quiz

Complete the following 15 multiple choice questions.

1. What is the preferred pH for detergents used for most cleaning processes?
   a. Low pH
   b. High pH
   c. Neutral pH
   d. It depends on the water temperature and exposure time

2. Which of the following statements about the use of mechanical washers is NOT true?
   a. Multi-level trays should be separated
   b. Trays with lids should be opened
   c. Instruments should be disassembled and opened
   d. All items should be washed on the same cycle

3. Water must be degassed each time the ultrasonic cleaner's tank is changed, because
   a. excess bubbles from filling reduce the energy of the cavitation process.
   b. excess bubbles reduce the effectiveness of the detergent.
   c. excess bubbles decrease the temperature of the tank.
   d. excess bubbles make it difficult to see items being cleaned.

4. Written cleaning instructions for surgical instruments should be provided by
   a. the mechanical washer manufacturer.
   b. the device manufacturer.
   c. the detergent manufacturer.
   d. the healthcare facility.

5. Pyrogens
   a. are fever-producing substances.
   b. are microorganisms that have survived sterilization.
   c. cause Creutzfeldt-Jakob disease.
   d. are soil particles.

6. Untreated water
   a. increases the likelihood of mineral scale deposits.
   b. decreases the likelihood of mineral scale deposits.
   c. is recommended to be used during the detergent cycle.
   d. is used for the final rinse process.

7. These are used to breakdown fatty tissue on instruments.
   a. Protease enzymes
   b. Lipase enzymes
   c. Amylase enzymes
   d. Neutral pH cleaners

8. Instrument lubrication is performed
   a. immediately before use.
   b. after sterilization.
   c. after cleaning.
   d. before cleaning.

115

9. To prevent coagulation of proteins, instruments should be pre-rinsed using
    a. cool water.
    b. warm water.
    c. a neutral detergent.
    d. a disinfectant rinse.

10. Detergents used in mechanical cleaners should be
    a. low alkaline.
    b. low acid.
    c. low temperature.
    d. low foaming.

11. Instruments should be cleaned using a
    a. circular motion.
    b. to and fro motion.
    c. stiff metal brush.
    d. water spray.

12. Powered surgical instruments
    a. cannot be immersed.
    b. can be immersed.
    c. should be cleaned at the point of use.
    d. should be cleaned using a mechanical washer.

13. The decontamination area should have
    a. negative air flow in relation to the other areas of the department.
    b. positive air flow in relation to the other areas of the department.
    c. 15 air exchanges per hour.
    d. positive air flow with 15 exchanges per hour.

14. The temperature in the decontamination area should be between
    a. 55 to 60 degrees Fahrenheit.
    b. 58 to 62 degrees Fahrenheit.
    c. 60 to 65 degrees Fahrenheit.
    d. 65 to 70 degrees Fahrenheit.

15. Rigid container filter retention plates should be
    a. removed from the container and lid and cleaned separately.
    b. manually cleaned and attached to the lid for mechanical cleaning.
    c. left attached to the lid during the cleaning process.
    d. none of the above.

Chapter 9: Disinfection Review Quiz

Complete the following 15 multiple choice and true/false questions.

1. This low-level disinfectant is incompatible with soap.
    a. Alcohol
    b. Phenol
    c. Quaternary ammonium compounds
    d. Ortho-phthalaldehyde

2. When using glutaraldehyde, technicians should always wear latex gloves for protection.
    a. True
    b. False

3. When using high-level disinfectants it is important to remember they may be deactivated by
    a. dilution.
    b. organic matter.
    c. time.
    d. all the above.

4. In an automated washer the key source of disinfection is
    a. hydrogen peroxide.
    b. water temperature.
    c. heat.
    d. disinfecting detergent.

5. The use of test strips to test the minimum effective concentration in high-level disinfection solutions is required
    a. weekly, preferably daily.
    b. daily.
    c. each time the solution will be used.
    d. only when manual soaking systems are used.

6. The use of heat to kill all microorganisms, except spores, is called
    a. sterilization.
    b. thermal disinfection.
    c. high-level disinfection.
    d. mechanical disinfection.

7. These chemicals are used on animate (living tissue) to slow the growth of microorganisms.
    a. Glutaraldehydes
    b. Disinfectants
    c. Halogens
    d. Antiseptics

8. Items that are introduced directly into the bloodstream or other normally sterile areas of the body are classified as
   a. critical items.
   b. semi-critical items.
   c. non-critical items.
   d. equipment.

9. The process by which all forms of microorganisms are completely destroyed is
   a. high-level disinfection.
   b. thermal disinfection.
   c. sterilization.
   d. chemical disinfection.

10. Iodophors are a member of this chemical family.
    a. Halogens
    b. Quaternary ammonium compounds
    c. Alcohol
    d. Phenolics

11. Phenolics are classified as
    a. intermediate to low-level disinfectants.
    b. intermediate to high-level disinfectants.
    c. high-level disinfectants.
    d. sterilants.

12. Which of the following are classified as high-level disinfectants?
    a. Glutaraldehyde and phenolics
    b. Glutaraldehyde and ortho-phthalaldehydes
    c. Quaternary ammonium compounds and phenolics
    d. Halogens and ortho-phthalaldehydes

13. Thermal disinfection is accomplished using
    a. heated chemicals.
    b. heated glurataldehyde.
    c. prolonged high pressure steam.
    d. heat.

14. How long must alcohol remain in wet contact with an item to achieve a reasonable level of disinfection?
    a. One to two minutes
    b. Two to three minutes
    c. Five to 10 minutes
    d. 10 to 20 minutes

15. Which of the following would be the best choice for high-level disinfection of instruments?
    a. Phenolics
    b. Chlorine
    c. Iodophors
    d. Ortho-phthalaldehydes

Chapter 10: Surgical Instrumentation Review Quiz

Indicate whether each of the following eight statements is true or false.

1. Microgrind or supercut scissors are usually identified with a black handle.
   a. True
   b. False

2. Stainless steel jaw needle holders last longer than tungsten carbide jaw needle holders.
   a. True
   b. False

3. The place where the two parts of a ring handled instrument meet and pivot is called the box lock.
   a. True
   b. False

4. Instruments are heat treated to give their surface a mirror (shiny) finish.
   a. True
   b. False

5. Tissue forceps have teeth.
   a. True
   b. False

6. During instrument manufacture the process of passivation helps build a protective chromium oxide layer on each instrument's surface.
   a. True
   b. False

7. The part of a hemostat that locks and holds it in position is called the box lock.
   a. True
   b. False

8. After applying instrument identification tape, instruments should be autoclaved to help the tape bond to the instrument.
   a. True
   b. False

Complete the following seven multiple choice questions.

9. Instrument marking tape should be wrapped approximately _____ around the instrument.
   a. 1.5 times
   b. two times
   c. 2.5 times
   d. three times

10. An osteotome is
    a. used to cut or shave bone.
    b. a retractor.
    c. a hemostatic forceps.
    d. used to dissect soft tissue.

11. The purpose of a suction stylet is to
    a. unclog the suction during surgery.
    b. clean the suction in the decontamination area.
    c. facilitate the sterilization process.
    d. provide a measuring guide for the surgeon.

12. Kerrison/laminectomy rongeurs should be tested using
    a. tissue paper.
    b. a plastic dowel rod.
    c. rubber testing material.
    d. an index card.

13. Scissors with tungsten carbide cutting edges are usually identified by
    a. black handles.
    b. silver handles.
    c. gold handles.
    d. the letters "TC".

14. The best way to clean a suction lumen is
    a. using running warm water.
    b. using the proper sized brush.
    c. soaking in an enzyme solution for three minutes.
    d. using the appropriate stylet.

15. To properly test the sharpness of scissors four inches or less use
    a. yellow test material.
    b. red test material.
    c. an index cart.
    d. orange test material.

Chapter 11: Complex Surgical Instruments Review Quiz

Complete the following 10 multiple choice questions.

1. The first step to inspect the insulation of a laparoscopic instrument is to
    a. check the collar at the distal tip.
    b. try to slide the insulation back.
    c. check the handle for chipping or cracking.
    d. visually check the instrument's shaft.

2. Which of the following steps happens first when processing flexible endoscopes?
    a. Leak-testing
    b. High-level disinfecting/sterilizing
    c. Manual cleaning
    d. Drying

3. Which of the following should be used to thoroughly rinse (remove) all traces of disinfectant from an endoscope's channels?
    a. Forced air
    b. Water containing approved sterilant
    c. Treated water
    d. A heated glutaraldehyde

4. The purpose of using a decontamination battery or hose when cleaning powered surgical instruments is
    a. to keep fluid from entering the unit.
    b. to keep functioning batteries and cords clean.
    c. to prevent electrical shock.
    d. to test the unit while cleaning.

5. Endoscopes are often processed in a mechanical unit called
    a. an ultrasonic cleaner.
    b. a washer-decontaminator.
    c. a flush-pulse endoscope reprocessor.
    d. an automatic endoscope reprocessor.

6. The endoscope that would be dispensed for a procedure that required visualization of the lower part of the large intestine would be a
    a. colonoscope.
    b. sigmoidoscope.
    c. gastroscope.
    d. ureteroscope.

7. Loaner instruments should
    a. be decontaminated if they appear soiled upon arrival.
    b. be sterilized using a low temperature process.
    c. be decontaminated before use.
    d. should not be used.

8. Information regarding cleaning processes for endoscopes should be provided by
    a. the Society of Gastroenterology Nurses and Associates.
    b. the Association for Professionals in Infection Control and Epidemiology.
    c. the instrument manufacturer.
    d. the Operating Room staff.

9. Which of the following statements about endoscopes is true?
    a. Not all endoscopes can be processed in an automatic endoscope reprocessor.
    b. Ultrasonic cleaning is the process of choice for endoscopes.
    c. Flexible endoscopes are not easily damaged.
    d. All endoscopes should be steam sterilized.

10. Electronic testing of laparoscopic insulation should be done
    a. in the decontamination area prior to cleaning.
    b. in the clean assembly area prior to set assembly.
    c. at the factory or onsite repair unit.
    d. in the Operating Room at the end of the procedure.

Indicate whether each of the following five statements is true or false.

11. Loaner instrumentation can cause receiving challenges.
    a. True
    b. False

12. Flexible endoscopes that fail a leak test may continue to be used until the break/hole impacts the scope's function.
    a. True
    b. False

13. All flexible endoscopes have internal channels.
    a. True
    b. False

14. After use, loaner instrumentation must be decontaminated before it is shipped out.
    a. True
    b. False

15. The biggest advantage to battery-powered surgical instruments is that they can be immersed for cleaning.
    a. True
    b. False

Chapter 12: Assembly and Packaging Review Quiz

Complete the following seven multiple choice questions.

1. The U.S. Food and Drug Administration classifies sterilization packaging as a
   a. Class I Medical Device
   b. Class II Medical Device
   c. Class III Medical Device
   d. Class IV Medical Device

2. Which of the following is NOT an acceptable sterilization packaging material?
   a. Muslin
   b. Barrier cloth
   c. Canvas
   d. Twills

3. Count sheets
   a. describe each instrument in detail.
   b. are used only for Operating Room trays and large procedure packs.
   c. provide a detailed list of tray contents.
   d. include manufacturer's Instructions for Use information.

4. When arranging paper/plastic pouches in the sterilizer, the pouches should be arranged
   a. paper-to-plastic.
   b. paper-to-paper.
   c. plastic-to-plastic.
   d. flat.

5. The relative humidity of the Central Service prep and pack area should be
   a. less than 75%.
   b. 30% to 60%.
   c. 40% to 80%.
   d. less than 35%.

6. Some plastics including formulations of spun-bonded polyolefin are intended for use solely in these sterilization processes
   a. steam.
   b. ozone and hydrogen peroxide.
   c. liquid.
   d. gravity.

7. When placing hinged instruments in an instrument tray, you should
   a. lock the handles to prevent damage during sterilization.
   b. arrange the instruments in alphabetical order.
   c. arrange the instruments in the order of their use.
   d. unlock the handles and open the instruments.

Indicate whether each of the following eight statements is true or false.

8. Gauze squares are the wicking material of choice for instrument sets.
   a. True
   b. False

9. Temperatures in a sterile storage area should be 55°F to 60°F.
   a. True
   b. False

10. When placing instruments in a peel pack, the tips should always face the plastic side of the pack.
    a. True
    b. False

11. All rigid sterilization containers have tamper-evident seals.
    a. True
    b. False

12. Cellulose materials cannot be processed within ozone sterilizers.
    a. True
    b. False

13. Reusable textile packaging requires less labor than disposable packaging.
    a. True
    b. False

14. Using latex tubing to protect delicate instrumentation is the process of choice for items to be steam sterilized.
    a. True
    b. False

15. While the outside of all instruments must be dry before sterilization it is important to ensure all lumens are kept moist for sterilization.
    a. True
    b. False

Chapter 13: Point-of-Use Processing Review Quiz
Complete the following 10 multiple choice and true/false questions.

1. The process by which instruments are steam sterilized for immediate use is called
   a. emergency sterilization.
   b. immediate use steam sterilization.
   c. core sterilization.
   d. rapid reprocessing.

2. Items to be disinfected or sterilized at the point of use must be
   a. properly cleaned per Manufacturer's Instructions for Use.
   b. semi-critical devices.
   c. non-critical devices.
   d. heat sensitive.

3. The best way to transport items that have been processed using immediate use steam sterilization at the point of use is
   a. covered with a sterile towel.
   b. in a rigid container designed for immediate use steam sterilization.
   c. in a covered mesh bottom tray.
   d. in a kraft paper bag.

4. Before an item can be placed in a liquid chemical sterile processing system they must be
   a. heated.
   b. filled with air.
   c. sterilized.
   d. cleaned.

5. Which of the following statements about immediate use steam sterilization is true?
   a. It is the sterilization method of choice for metal instruments
   b. It is recommended to be used as a primary sterilization process by the Association for the Advancement of Medical Instrumentation and the Association of periOperative Registered Nurses
   c. It reduces turnaround time because cleaning is not required
   d. It should be used only when there is not time to process items using the wrapped method

6. Both the Association of periOperative Registered Nurses and The Joint Commission recommend that
   a. the use of immediate use steam sterilization be minimized or decreased.
   b. immediate use steam sterilization be performed in only one sterilizer per facility.
   c. healthcare facilities get U.S. Food and Drug Administration approval for immediate use steam sterilization.
   d. only Central Service technicians operate immediate use steam sterilizers.

7. Implantable devices
   a. should be immediate use steam sterilization in extended cycles.
   b. should only be sterilized using ethylene oxide.
   c. should not be immediate use steam sterilization sterilized unless there is a tracking system in place to trace the item to a patient.
   d. require double cycle sterilization to ensure sterility.

8. When transporting items that have been immediate use steam sterilized, it is required that
   a. they be transported in a metal container.
   b. they be transported to the patient area within five minutes of the completion of the sterilization cycle.
   c. they be allow to properly cooled before transport.
   d. they be transported in such a manner that reduces the potential for contamination.

9. When sterilizing items at the point of use, an abbreviated sterilization cycle may be used due to the urgent need for the instruments.
   a. True
   b. False

10. Immediate use steam sterilization documentation should include
    a. the name of the patient for which the items were sterilized.
    b. sterilizer number and cycle.
    c. name of the instrument sterilized.
    d. all the above.

Chapter 14: High-Temperature Sterilization Review Quiz

Complete the following 20 multiple choice and true/false questions.

1. When loading a steam sterilizer, basins should be
   a. placed in an upright position.
   b. loaded first.
   c. placed on edge.
   d. placed in a wire basket.

2. The higher the bioburden on an object
   a. the more difficult it will be to sterilize.
   b. the less time it will take to sterilize it.
   c. the more biological tests you will need in the load.
   d. the longer it will take to cool after sterilization.

3. When combining loads, hard goods should be placed on the top shelves to allow for more efficient removal of the condensate.
   a. True
   b. False

4. The steam sterilization process can be affected by the design of the medical device being sterilized.
   a. True
   b. False

5. Central Service technicians need to understand the anatomy of a steam sterilizer to
   a. know how to properly clean the chamber.
   b. understand how the sterilizer operates.
   c. understand how to test the thermostatic trap.
   d. know how to properly maintain the jacket.

6. The weakest part of a steam sterilizer is the
   a. jacket.
   b. gasket.
   c. door.
   d. thermostatic valve.

7. Three of the main phases of a terminal steam sterilizer cycle are
   a. gravity, exposure and exhaust.
   b. pre-vacuum, exposure and exhaust.
   c. exposure, exhaust and dry.
   d. conditioning, exposure and exhaust.

8. The most common reason for steam sterilization failure is
   a. lack of steam contact with the instrument.
   b. insufficient temperature.
   c. inadequate exposure time.
   d. drying issues.

9. The coolest place in a steam sterilizer is the
   a. gasket.
   b. thermostatic valve.
   c. jacket.
   d. chamber.

10. Steam flush pressure pulse sterilizers are a type of gravity sterilizers.
   a. True
   b. False

11. Factors that can cause sterilant contact failure with the instrument are
   a. cleaning, loosely packed load.
   b. conditioning, size and weight of the instrument.
   c. solid bottom containers, exposure time.
   d. crowded loads, clogged drain strainer.

12. One of the most frequent causes of a clogged drain screen is
   a. tape.
   b. wrapper particles.
   c. poor steam quality.
   d. malfunctioning baffle plate.

13. After sterilization the load contents may take two hours or more to cool.
   a. True
   b. False

14. Peel pouches should be placed _____ for sterilization.
   a. on edge, paper to plastic
   b. on edge, plastic to plastic
   c. placed flat with the plastic side up
   d. placed flat with the paper side up

15. Items with a standard steam sterilization cycle recommended by the manufacturer can be damaged if run in an extended cycle.
   a. True
   b. False

16. How frequently should a sterilizer's strainer be removed and cleaned?
   a. Daily
   b. After each use
   c. Once weekly
   d. Only when the machine's operating control gauge indicates cleaning is necessary

17. Immediate use steam sterilization is the process to sterilize trays for future use.
   a. True
   b. False

18. Wood products should be sterilized in an extended steam cycle.
    a. True
    (b.) False

19. When water is seen on the outside of a pack after sterilization the pack is considered safe to use if all other packs in the load are dry.
    a. True
    (b.) False

20. Packs that are improperly packaged or loaded on the sterilizer cart frequently become wet packs.
    (a) True
    b. False

Chapter 15: Low-Temperature Sterilization Review Quiz

Complete the following 10 multiple choice and true/false questions.

1. Woven reusable fabrics are the packaging products of choice for ozone sterilization.
   a. True
   b. False

2. Ethylene kills microorganisms by a process called oxidation.
   a. True
   b. False

3. Ethylene oxide, hydrogen peroxide and ozone sterilization process must all be monitored using chemical, physical and biological monitors.
   a. True
   b. False

4. Ethylene oxide, hydrogen peroxide and ozone sterilization can all use the same packaging materials.
   a. True
   b. False

5. Lumens should be moist when using hydrogen peroxide as a sterilizing agent.
   a. True
   b. False

6. Ethylene oxide is a toxic gas.
   a. True
   b. False

7. Cellulose-containing packaging materials are not compatible with hydrogen peroxide sterilization.
   a. True
   b. False

8. Information about a device's compatibility with a specific sterilization process should be obtained from the device's manufacturer.
   a. True
   b. False

9. An extended aeration cycle is required for items sterilized in ozone sterilization processes.
   a. True
   b. False

10. Permissible exposure levels for low-temperature sterilization methods are established by the
    a. U.S. Food and Drug Administration.
    b. Centers for Disease Control.
    c. Occupational Safety and Health Administration.
    d. Environmental Protection Agency.

Chapter 16: Sterile Storage and Transport Review Quiz

Complete the following 15 multiple choice and true/false questions.

1. The relative humidity of the Central Service sterile storage area should be
   a. less than 70%.
   b. less than 60%.
   c. less than 50%.
   d. less than 35%.

2. Temperatures in a sterile storage area should be 64⁰ to 75⁰ F.
   a. True
   b. False

3. Because of event-related shelf life, stock rotation is no longer necessary.
   a. True
   b. False

4. The sterile storage process starts
   a. when items are received in the decontamination area.
   b. after items are sterilized and cooled.
   c. when the sterilizer door is opened.
   d. when items are placed into the sterilizer.

5. Sterile storage areas should
   a. have positive airflow and at least 10 air exchanges per hour.
   b. have positive airflow and at least four air exchanges per hour.
   c. have negative airflow and at least 10 air exchanges per hour.
   d. have negative airflow and at least four air exchanges per hour.

6. Temperature and humidity levels in the sterile storage area should be checked and recorded at least weekly.
   a. True
   b. False

7. The shelving system of choice for the sterile storage area is
   a. closed.
   b. semi closed.
   c. open.
   d. tracked.

8. Trays which overhang shelving
   a. can become contaminated.
   b. are ok for rigid containers, but not for flat wrapped trays.
   c. is the appropriate way to store trays as it allows for the use of proper body mechanics when lifting heavy trays.
   d. none of the above.

9. The type of shelving that leaves packaging the most vulnerable is
    a. open.
    b. closed.
    c. semi closed.
    d. tracked.

10. The bottom shelf of any sterile storage system should be
    a. solid and eight to 10 inches from the floor.
    b. solid and two to four inches from the floor.
    c. cleaned weekly.
    d. wire and eight to 10 inches from the floor.

11. Sterile trays should
    a. not be touched until they are properly cooled.
    b. be lifted not dragged off the sterilizer cart.
    c. be checked to be sure the chemical indicators have turned the appropriate color.
    d. all the above.

12. Wrapped trays should not be stacked because
    a. the tray contents may be damaged.
    b. it can cause holes in the wrapper of the bottom tray.
    c. it will cause the shelving to bend.
    d. they will be more difficult to rotate.

13. Outside shipping containers
    a. should be removed prior to placing the items in storage.
    b. may be stored in the sterile storage area as long as they are not stored near the in-house sterilized items.
    c. make good storage containers to help keep items from falling from the shelves.
    d. all the above.

14. Event-related shelf life means items are safe until opened for use.
    a. True
    b. False

15. Sterilized packages may be jeopardized due to storage practices.
    a. True
    b. False

Chapter 17: Monitoring and Recordkeeping for Central Service Review Quiz

Complete the following 10 multiple choice and true/false questions.

1. Formal training should occur
    a. for new employees.
    b. at least monthly.
    c. for employees who move to a new positions.
    d. for new employees and those who move to new positions.

2. Monitoring records must be
    a. accurate.
    b. legible.
    c. complete.
    d. all the above.

3. Sterilizer load records should contain
    a. items and quantity sterilized.
    b. type of packaging used in the load.
    c. preventive maintenance dates.
    d. all the above.

4. External indicators can prove an item is sterile when the sterilization cycle is complete.
    a. True
    b. False

5. Temperature and humidity levels need to be monitored and recorded
    a. weekly, preferably daily.
    b. for each shift.
    c. at least daily.
    d. at least monthly.

6. The U.S. Food and Drug Administration Class II chemical indicator that is run daily in dynamic air removal sterilizers is called a
    a. process challenge device.
    b. external chemical indicator.
    c. biological indicator.
    d. Bowie-Dick test.

7. One type of formal monitoring is monitoring the department temperature and humidity levels.
    a. True
    b. False

8. A physical monitor on a washer-disinfector is the
    a. thermostatic valve.
    b. printout.
    c. biological test.
    d. all the above.

9. Cart washer screens should be cleaned at least
    a. daily.
    b. during each shift.
    c. weekly, preferably daily.
    d. monthly.

10. A biological indicator is called positive when
    a. the incubation process is complete.
    b. there is no growth in the ampule after incubation.
    c. there is growth in the ampule after incubation.
    d. prior to sterilization.

Chapter 18: Quality Assurance Review Quiz

Indicate whether each of the following 10 statements is true or false.

1. Quality requires the efforts and participation of everyone in the healthcare facility.
   a. **True**
   b. False

2. A failure mode and effects analysis tries to predict failures before they occur.
   a. **True**
   b. False

3. The International Standards Organization uses routine and unannounced inspections to monitor standards in healthcare facilities.
   a. True
   b. **False**

4. Quality processes are limited to administration and the risk management department.
   a. True
   b. **False**

5. Quality management is patient focused.
   a. **True**
   b. False

6. Providing quality products and services directly impacts patient outcomes.
   a. True
   b. **False**

7. Customer surveys are ineffective tools in establishing Central Service quality processes.
   a. **True**
   b. **False**

8. If everyone develops a quality-driven focus, written policies and procedures are not necessary in the Central Service department.
   a. True
   b. **False**

9. A root cause analysis is a proactive approach to quality.
   a. True
   b. **False**

10. Not following established policies and procedures will result in a lower quality program.
    a. **True**
    b. False

Chapter 19: Managing Inventory within the Central Service Department Review Quiz

Complete the following 10 multiple choice and true/false questions.

1. Which of the following systems provides supplies and instruments for individual surgical procedures?
   a. Exchange cart
   b. Periodic automated replenishment system
   c. Case cart
   d. Requisition

2. The inventory system that stocks supplies by established stock levels is called
   a. a periodic automated replenishment system.
   b. case cart.
   c. an ADT system.
   d. exchange system.

3. The inventory system that uses two identical carts to facilitate supply replenishment is called the
   a. case cart system.
   b. exchange cart system.
   c. periodic automated replenishment system.
   d. requisition system.

4. Automated supply replenishment systems are
   a. no longer used.
   b. used only in surgery.
   c. difficult to manage.
   d. computerized.

5. The movement of supplies throughout the healthcare facility is called
   a. distribution.
   b. inventory management.
   c. case cart system.
   d. procurement.

6. Operational supplies are supplies that are dispensed for patient care.
   a. True
   b. False

7. Supplies such as disposable wraps are called
   a. consumable.
   b. capital supplies.
   c. patient care supplies.
   d. non-refundable supplies.

8. Capital equipment items are
   a. usually used for patient care.
   b. items with a lower purchase cost.
   c. items with a higher purchase cost.
   d. purchased, stored, consumed and reordered.

9. The following symbolizes

   a. product lot number.
   b. use by date.
   c. single-use item (do not reuse).
   d. product manufacture date.

10. The following symbolizes

   a. product lot number.
   b. use by date.
   c. single-use item (do not reuse).
   d. product manufacture date.

Chapter 20: The Role of Central Service in Ancillary Department Support Review Quiz

Complete the following 15 multiple choice questions.

1. Technicians in the _____ department perform safety inspections and functional tests on equipment.
   a. Materiel Management
   b. infection control
   c. Biomedical engineering
   d. facilities and maintenance

2. When patient equipment enters a healthcare facility, it must be safety checked by a_____ before it is cleared for patient use.
   a. Biomedical technician
   b. infection control committee member
   c. Central Service technician
   d. Central Service director

3. Which of the following requires that preventive maintenance standards be established for medical equipment?
   a. Occupational Safety and Health Administration
   b. The Joint Commission
   c. Association for the Advancement of Medical Instrumentation
   d. National Institute for Occupational Safety and Health

4. All patient care equipment that was dispensed for use must be Considered _____ and handled as such, regardless of its appearance.
   a. sterile
   b. clean
   c. contaminated
   d. visibly soiled

5. Which of the following common items of patient care equipment limits the development of deep vein thrombosis and peripheral edema in immobile patients?
   a. Respirator
   b. Intermittent suction device
   c. Sequential compression unit
   d. Defibrillator

6. Disposable components such as pads and tubing on patient care equipment should be
   a. discarded at the point of use.
   b. be reprocessed for re-use.
   c. discarded during preventive maintenance.
   d. removed in the biomedical engineering department.

7. Equipment should be inspected for obvious hazards such as cracked or frayed electrical cords
    a. only by trained biomedical engineering technicians.
    b. only during preventive maintenance activities.
    c. only when there are complaints from user department personnel.
    d. whenever the equipment is inspected in Central Service.

8. If an equipment malfunction causes harm to patients, it should be
    a. discarded immediately.
    b. sent to the manufacturer for repairs.
    c. sequestered for inspection by Occupational Safety and Health Administration personnel.
    d. returned immediately to the biomedical department.

9. Patient care equipment should be stored in a _____ condition.
    a. "ready to dispense"
    b. "ready to clean"
    c. "ready to inspect"
    d. "ready to sterilize"

10. Patient care equipment is typically stored
    a. in the Biomedical engineering department.
    b. in patient units.
    c. in the Central Service department.
    d. in sterile storage areas of the Materiel Management department.

11. The _____ requires that the healthcare facility report malfunctions of medical devices that have contributed to patient injury, illness and/or death to the manufacturer and the U.S. Food and Drug Administration.
    a. Occupational Safety and Health Administration Patient Safety Act
    b. Safe Medical Devices Act
    c. Environmental Protection Agency Patient Security Act
    d. U.S. Food and Drug Administration Equipment Notification Act

12. Which of the following statements is correct?
    a. Patient care equipment tracking requires a computer
    b. Patient care equipment should only be tracked if it has a value in excess of an amount specified by the facility
    c. Tracking patient care equipment can prevent equipment shortages
    d. Patient care equipment must only be tracked if its usage will be charged to patients

13. Equipment leasing and rental differ in that
    a. leasing involves purchase; rental does not require ownership.
    b. equipment rental is usually done on a shorter-term basis than equipment leasing.
    c. equipment leasing involves the most expensive equipment; equipment rental involves less expensive equipment.
    d. equipment leasing is an operating expense; equipment rental does not have cost implications.

14. Preventive maintenance is
    a. performed when a piece of equipment injures a patient.
    b. designed to identify potential problems before they occur.
    c. performed when a user unit notices a problem.
    d. done by Central Service before equipment is dispensed.

15. The decision to use reusable or disposable instruments in procedure trays is determined by
    a. where the instruments will be used.
    b. the Infection Prevention department.
    c. several factors including physician preference, storage and cost.
    d. amount of items to be used and delivery schedule.

Chapter 21: The Role of Information Technology in Central Service Review Quiz

Complete the following 15 multiple choice and true/false questions.

1. In addition to providing financial and operational management, information technology and systems are used to help ensure patient safety.
   - a. True
   - b. False

2. Information technology is often the cornerstone of initiatives to transform healthcare.
   - a. True
   - b. False

3. Which of the following is NOT a result of computer integration?
   - a. Eliminating redundant entry of information
   - b. Promotes efficiency
   - c. Automatically provides critical update to industry standards
   - d. Reduced inaccurate and conflicting information

4. Patient census information used in Central Service is obtained from the electronic health record.
   - a. True
   - b. False

5. Computer supply chain management systems are used to monitor facility assets.
   - a. True
   - b. False

6. Tracking individual instruments is important to help ensure specific instruments are kept with a specific set.
   - a. True
   - b. False

7. Which of the following is NOT a reason for tracking supplies, equipment and instruments?
   - a. Monitoring item usage
   - b. Ensuring that items can be quickly located
   - c. Meeting Centers for Disease Control and Occupational Safety and Health Administration requirements
   - d. Assisting with quality processes

8. Which of the following tracking methods provides real-time information?
    a. Radio frequency identification tags
    b. Laser-etched bar codes
    c. Standard bar codes
    d. Dot matrix applications

9. Point-of-use computing
    a. is impossible in Central Service because of infection control requirements.
    b. provides no benefit to the Central Service department.
    c. moves computers into Central Service work areas.
    d. eliminates data entry jobs.

10. Which of the following is NOT a feature of an instrument tracking system?
    a. Productivity information
    b. Financial data
    c. Quality assurance information
    d. Product updates and recall information

11. Computerized tracking systems are fast, but manual tracking systems are more effective for tracking.
    a. True
    b. False

12. Once a tracking system is implemented, there is generally no need to update system information.
    a. True
    b. False

13. At this time, tracking systems are unable to track worker productivity information.
    a. True
    b. False

14. Tracking systems can help manage preventive maintenance schedules.
    a. True
    b. False

15. Most Central Service departments employ some sort of automated information management system.
    a. True
    b. False

Chapter 22: Safety and Risk Management for Central Service Review Quiz

Complete the following 15 multiple choice and true/false questions.

1. Risk management programs are designed to prevent accidents and injury.
   - a. True
   - b. False

2. Which of the following is NOT a component of risk management?
   - a. Injury prevention
   - b. Claims management
   - c. Staff management
   - d. Risk assessment

3. Which of the following is NOT considered one of the three occupational hazards?
   - a. Physical hazards
   - b. Ergonomic hazards
   - c. Biological hazards
   - d. Chemical hazards

4. Information about chemical or hazardous substances must be available to all employees.
   - a. True
   - b. False

5. Healthcare facilities are required by the _____ to provide adequate ventilation systems, personal protective equipment and safe work operating procedures?
   - a. Environmental Protection Agency
   - b. U.S. Food and Drug Administration
   - c. Occupational Safety and Health Administration
   - d. Centers for Medicare and Medicaid Services

6. Time-weighted average is defined as the amount of a substance you can be exposed to over an eight-hour day.
   - a. True
   - b. False

7. The process of changing work or working conditions to reduce physical stress is
   - a. called ergonomics.
   - b. an employee injury reduction plan.
   - c. the Occupational Safety and Health Administration Workers' Rights Program.
   - d. the Occupational Safety and Health Administration Risk Management Program.

8. The key to working safely is keeping your work area organized.
   - a. True
   - b. False

9. When you cannot see what is in a sink or basin you should
    a. drain the sink or basin.
    b. use a sponge forceps to grasp items.
    c. have someone help you determine what is in the sink or basin.
    d. all the above.

10. Which of the following is NOT required for sharps safety?
    a. Dispose of all single use sharps in an appropriate container
    b. Sharp ends should be pointed away from anyone's body during transport
    c. Wash all disposable sharps before discarding them
    d. All the above

11. The level of exposure to a harmful substance when an employer must take required precautions to protect the worker.
    a. Time-weighted average
    b. Short-term excursion limit
    c. Permissible exposure limit
    d. Action level

12. Ergonomic injuries
    a. are not a concern for Central Service employees.
    b. are rare in today's work environment.
    c. are a risk factor for persons who perform repetitive or physical work.
    d. happen only in the office setting.

13. Secondary containers of chemicals
    a. must be labeled with a copy of the original manufacturer's label or a generic label that identifies hazard warnings and directions.
    b. must be labeled with a permanent marker and must state the chemical's name and designated storage location.
    c. secondary containers of chemicals are not allowed in healthcare facilities.
    d. there are no restrictions for secondary container labels at this time.

14. Safety data sheets are provided by the
    a. Occupational Safety and Health Administration.
    b. U.S. Food and Drug Administration.
    c. Risk Management department.
    d. product manufacturer.

15. A molecular reaction that creates an uncontrolled release of energy is called
    a. combustion.
    b. polymerization.
    c. vapor density.
    d. fire.

Chapter 23: Success through Communication Review Quiz

Complete the following 15 multiple choice questions.

1. Which of the following is an example of communication?
   a. Spoken word
   b. Written word
   c. Non-verbal expressions
   d. All of the above

2. Central Service technicians who do not think they are being treated appropriately by their employer should
   a. find another job.
   b. discuss the problem with their workplace peers.
   c. discuss the situation with their supervisor.
   d. accept the situation as "the way things are done" at the facility.

3. Behavior relating to what is "right and wrong" relative to the standards of conduct for your profession are called
   a. ethical behavior.
   b. moral behavior.
   c. legal behavior.
   d. personal behavior.

4. A step in communication that occurs when a listener asks a question is called
   a. stereotyping.
   b. feedback.
   c. communication looping.
   d. halo interpretation.

5. This process allows a person to understand someone else's needs.
   a. Communication
   b. Human relations
   c. Feedback
   d. Moral behavior

6. When speaking, you should
   a. be influenced by the listener's emotions.
   b. concentrate on the listener rather than oneself.
   c. concentrate on yourself rather than the listener.
   d. use technical jargon to impress the listener.

7. Which of the following basic listening tactics is most useful?
   a. Try to listen only for specific facts
   b. Ignore any non-verbal communication "sent" by the speaker
   c. Focus on the delivery of the message rather than its content
   d. None of the above

8. The ability to use information gained from words or body language to interact with others.
    a. Communication
    b. Human relations
    c. Teamwork
    d. Mentoring

9. Which of the following is the most important factor necessary for teamwork?
    a. Attitude
    b. Promptness
    c. Loyalty
    d. Cooperation

10. Which of the following statements is correct?
    a. Informal work groups are "bad" for the organization
    b. Informal work groups develop an informal communication system called the grapevine
    c. A task group is an example of an informal group
    d. Employees can only be members of one formal group at a time

11. A group of employees from different departments within the healthcare facility that work together to solve operating problems is called a
    a. decision-making team.
    b. multi-dimensional team.
    c. cross-functional team.
    d. management/sub-management team.

12. Which of the following is true about a valuing diversity effort?
    a. It "happens" because top-level officials require it
    b. It occurs because a Central Service director desires it
    c. It is a "program" in which a committee "decides what to do"
    d. None of the above

13. Coaching is an example of
    a. informal communication.
    b. discipline.
    c. formal communication.
    d. Mentoring.

14. Knowing what is expected and consistently meeting those expectations is part of
    a. effective communications.
    b. ethical behavior.
    c. job success.
    d. professional behavior.

15. When Central Service technicians have internet access at work
    a. it should be used for work-related purposes only.
    b. it may be used for any purposes as long as it doesn't interfere with work.
    c. it should only be used during break time.
    d. they should follow the facility's policy.

Chapter 24: Personal and Professional Development for Central Services Review Quiz

Complete the following 10 multiple choice and true/false questions.

1. Which of the following is an open-ended question?
   a. "How long have you worked here?"
   b. "Do you like your job?"
   c. "What problems do you most frequently encounter on the job?"
   d. "What is the name of the Central Service director?"

2. Personal development improves your employability skills.
   a. True
   b. False

3. When setting personal goals you should set goals that are
   a. quickly attainable.
   b. attainable within five years then set new goals.
   c. attainable, then build on those successes.
   d. specific to your current position and education.

4. Professional development helps give you the information and experience needed to progress in your career.
   a. True
   b. False

5. Teaching others increases your understanding of the standards.
   a. True
   b. False

6. Planning and reviewing your goals will help identify activities to help you meet those goals.
   a. True
   b. False

7. Resources found online have already been determined to be valid before they are posted online.
   a. True
   b. False

8. Steps toward attaining professional goals in Central Service include
   a. obtaining certification.
   b. attending educational conferences.
   c. participating in professional groups.
   d. all the above.

9. One important step in preparing for an interview is
    a. reviewing the certification exam questions.
    b. developing a written response to application questions.
    c. anticipating possible interview questions.
    d. all the above.

10. On the job relationships do NOT change when one team member has been promoted.
    a. True
    b. False

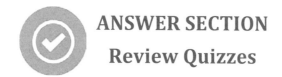

ANSWER SECTION
Review Quizzes

Chapter 1: Introduction to Central Service Review Quiz

1. Soiled instruments and other items are received in the _____ area of the Central Service department.
   c. *decontamination*   *(10)*

2. The first step in the sterilization process is
   d. *cleaning.*   *(10)*

3. Central Service technicians must wear special attire referred to as _____ to minimize their exposure to bloodborne pathogens and other contaminants.
   a. *PPE*   *(11)*

4. Instrument sets and other required instrumentation needed for all scheduled procedures for an entire day are usually pulled (collected)
   b. *the day or evening before they will be used.*   *(13)*

5. The use of analytical skills to solve problems and make decisions is a component of which of the following knowledge and skills dimensions?
   c. *Employability skills*   *(16)*

6. Healthcare-associated infections are
   d. *infections which occur in the course of being treated in a healthcare facility.*   *(18)*

7. The human resources tool that defines job duties performed by persons in specific positions is called a
   d. *job description.*   *(18)*

8. In the future, which of the following will more frequently become a requirement for working in a Central Service department?
   c. *Formal education*   *(19)*

9. While items may be dispensed to all areas of a facility, the major focus of the sterile storage personnel is
   d. *the Operating Room.*   *(13)*

10. Which of the following is NOT a growing trend in Central Service?
    a. *Decentralization of Central Service responsibilities*   *(9)*

Chapter 2: Medical Terminology for Central Service Technicians Review Quiz

1. Knowing and understanding medical terminology helps technicians
   c. *understand what is asked when a request is made.*   *(22)*

2. The majority of medical terms are of either _____ or _____ origin.
   b. *Greek or Latin*   *(23)*

3. Which of the following tells the primary meaning of a word?
     b. *Root word element*

(23)

4. The purpose of a combining vowel is to
     c. *ease pronunciation of a word.*   (24)

5. The last word element in a medical term is the
     c. *suffix.*   (24)

6. The term *itis* means
     b. *inflammation.*   (27)

7. The term *ectomy* means
     b. *surgical removal.*   (28)

8. The term *oscopy* means
     a. *visual examination.*   (28)

9. Arthroscopy means
     a. *visual exam of a joint.*   (28)

10. The term *ostomy*
     b. *is a suffix.*   (28)

11. The suffix *-tome* means a
     d. *cutting instrument.*   (29)

12. *Plasty* is a
     c. *suffix meaning surgical restoration.*   (29)

13. The word *laminectomy* means
     b. *removal of part of a lamina.*   (28)

14. Which of the following means *beside* or *near*?
     a. *Para*   (25)

15. Which of the following surgical abbreviations might be used relating to a
    fractured bone?
     c. *ORIF*   (35)

16. The term *intercostal* means
     d. *between the ribs.*   (32)

17. The term *hypo* means
     c. *below.*   (32)

18. The term *septorhinoplasty* means
     b. *surgical repair of the nose.*   (25)

19. Encephalopathy is a/an
     a. *disease of the brain.*   (27)

20. Lithotripsy means
     c. *crushing of a stone.*   (31)

1. This system gives the body shape and support.
    c. *Skeletal system*   *(43)*

2. This tissue acts as a cushion between the bones to prevent them from rubbing together.
    c. *Cartilage*   *(44)*

3. These muscles control involuntary movements like breathing, digestion, etc.
    a. *Smooth*   *(48)*

4. This surgical procedure consists of removing an ear bone that has thickened and no longer transmits sound waves and replacing it with an artificial implant to improve hearing.
    b. *Stapedectomy*   *(53)*

5. More than 55% of blood is made up of this yellowish liquid.
    d. *Plasma*   *(63)*

6. An organ the filters the blood to remove amino acids and neutralize some harmful toxins.
    c. *Liver*   *(58)*

7. This surgical procedure removes the uterus.
    b. *Hysterectomy*   *(56)*

8. This gland stimulates body growth.
    d. *Pituitary*   *(54)*

9. This is the lining of the uterus.
    b. *Endometrium*   *(55)*

10. This surgical procedure removes tissue or displaced bone from the wrist area to release pressure on the median nerve.
    a. *Carpal tunnel repair*   *(52)*

11. The largest part of the human brain is the
    c. *cerebrum.*   *(49)*

12. This surgical procedure is the relocation of an undescended testicle.
    c. *Orchiopexy*   *(56)*

13. The throat is also called the
    d. *pharynx.*   *(59)*

14. This surgical procedure is the removal of the gall bladder.
    a. *Cholecystectomy*   *(62)*

15. The hip joint is an example of a
    b. *ball and socket joint.*   *(44)*

16. This tissue covers the body's external surface.
    a. Epithelial tissue   (43)

17. The brain center of a cell is the
    c. nucleus.   (42)

18. Cartilage is replaced by bone through a process called
    a. ossification.   (44)

19. The white portion of the eye is called the
    d. sclera.   (50)

20. This is referred to as the voice box.
    b. Larynx   (59)

Chapter 4: Microbiology for Central Service Technicians Review Quiz   page reference

1. Healthy people do not harbor or transmit bacteria.
    b. False   (70)

2. Anaerobic bacteria require free oxygen to live.
    b. False   (72)

3. Viruses are larger than bacteria.
    b. False   (78)

4. The spore is the control unit of a cell.
    b. False   (71)

5. Staphylococcus is classified as a gram-positive bacteria.
    a. True   (74)

6. All microorganisms are harmful to humans.
    b. False   (71)

7. Spores help some microorganisms survive in adverse conditions.
    a. True   (73)

8. All bacteria require the same conditions to live and grow.
    b. False   (75)

9. Psychrophiles grow best in warm temperatures.
    b. False   (75)

10. When cleaning prion-contaminated instruments no special cleaning procedures are
    required, only following standard cleaning protocols and the manufacturer's Instructions
    for Use is necessary.
    b. False   (81)

11. Microorganisms reproduce by a process called
  b. *binary fission.*   *(76)*

12. Bacteria that cause disease are called
  c. *pathogens.*   *(71)*

13. The part of a cell that controls cell function is the
  b. *nucleus.*   *(71)*

14. The virus that causes hepatitis B is transmitted by
  b. *blood.*   *(79)*

15. _____ is an example of a fungus.
  c. *Athlete's foot*   *(80)*

Chapter 5: Regulations and Standards Review Quiz   *page reference*

1. Agency which may intervene in a matter of worker protection even if there are no specific regulations covering the situation.
  a. *Occupational Safety and Health Administration*   *(93)*

2. Regulations under the Clean Air Act are administered by
  c. *Environmental Protection Agency*   *(92)*

3. The agency which imposes very strict labeling requirements on manufacturers of disinfectants used by Central Service departments.
  c. *Environmental Protection Agency*   *(92)*

4. Healthcare regulations and standards establish
  a. *minimal levels of quality and safety.*   *(86)*

5. Chemical indicators are classified as
  b. *FDA Class II medical devices.*   *(87)*

6. Heart valves and pacemakers are examples of
  c. *FDA Class III medical devices.*   *(87)*

7. Under current regulations, who is required to report suspected medical device-related deaths to the U.S. Food and Drug Administration?
  c. *All of the above*   *(88)*

8. Standards and regulations help set levels of _____ in our departments.
  d. *both quality and safety*   *(86)*

9. Medical device reporting is regulated by the
  d. *U.S. Food and Drug Administration*   *(88)*

10. The Department of Transportation enforces statutes relating to the
  b. *transportation of unclean, damaged flexible endoscopes.*   *(91)*

11. Sometimes state or local regulations differ from Federal regulations and when that happens, the most stringent regulations apply.
    a. *True* *(95)*

12. Following the Occupational Safety and Health Administration's regulations for wearing personal protective equipment in the Central Service decontamination area is optional.
    b. *False* *(95)*

13. Third-party reprocessors are regulated by the U.S. Food and Drug Administration.
    a. *True* *(90)*

14. Recommendations regarding sterilization practices are provided by the Association for the Advancement of Medical Instrumentation.
    a. *True* *(95)*

15. The American National Standards Institute is a voluntary association dedicated to infection control and prevention.
    b. *False* *(96)*

16. Failure to receive accreditation from The Joint Commission can result in the loss of Medicare and Medicaid payments.
    a. *True* *(97)*

17. The Society of Gastroenterology Nurses and Associates is a source for information about the proper processing of flexible endoscopes.
    a. *True* *(98)*

18. Class III medical devices are identified as high risk.
    a. *True* *(87)*

19. Reuse of single use medical devices is less regulated now than it was in the 1990's.
    b. *False* *(90)*

20. The U.S. Food and Drug Administration recalls may be either mandatory or voluntary.
    a. *True* *(89)*

Chapter 6: Infection Prevention and Control Review Quiz   *page reference*

1. Each year, approximately _____ patients develop a healthcare-associated infection.
    c. *700,000* *(102)*

2. Jewelry should NOT be worn in the Central Service department work areas because they
    a. *harbor bacteria.* *(107)*

3. During handwashing, hands should be lathered and scrubbed for at least
    b. *20 seconds* *(105)*

4. To protect themselves from splashes and spills, Central Service technicians assigned to the decontamination area should wear
    c. *fluid-resistant gowns.*   *(108)*

5. The main theory of standard precautions is
    d. *to treat all human blood and bodily fluids as infectious.*   *(103)*

6. Which of the following is NOT a requirement of the Occupational Safety and Health Administration Bloodborne Pathogen Standard?
    c. *Keep biohazard areas locked*   *(111)*

7. The only way to interrupt the transmission of a causative agent is to
    c. *eliminate it.*   *(115)*

8. Departmental dress codes applies to
    a. *everyone entering the Central Service department.*   *(108)*

9. Inanimate objects that can transmit bacteria are called
    b. *fomites.*   *(113)*

10. Floors in the Central Service department should be
    a. *wet-mopped daily.*   *(114)*

11. The absence of microorganisms that cause disease is called
    c. *asepsis.*   *(104)*

12. Know what is dirty, know what is clean, know what is sterile. Keep these three conditions separate and remedy contamination immediately are known as
    a. *the principles of asepsis.*   *(104)*

13. What color should biohazard labels/signs be?
    a. *Red/orange*   *(111)*

14. The decontamination area of the Central Service department should have
    a. *negative air flow.*   *(112)*

15. Which of these traffic control/dress code requirements applies to the clean assembly area of Central Service?
    c. *Semi restricted*   *(110)*

1. Items that have been used in patient care should be considered contaminated.
    *   *a.   True*   *(126)*

2. If soiled items are held in user units before pick up for processing, they must be kept at the patient's bedside until Central Service collects them.
    *   *b.   False*   *(121)*

3. To help prevent the growth of biofilm, soil on used instruments should be allowed to dry.
    *   *b.   False*   *(126)*

4. Users are responsible to notify Central Service if they discover instruments or equipment that need repair.
    *   *a.   True*   *(124)*

5. It is acceptable to transport soiled and clean items at the same time in the same cart if they are placed on separate shelves.
    *   *b.   False*   *(125)*

6. When moving transport carts throughout the healthcare facility, Central Service technicians must always yield right of way to patients and visitors.
    *   *a.   True*   *(126)*

7. Failure to perform soiled pick-up rounds as scheduled can lead to instrument and equipment shortages.
    *   *a.   True*   *(126)*

8. Everyone who may transport contaminated items must be trained in safe handling procedures.
    *   *a.   True*   *(125)*

9. When it is necessary to transport soiled items between facilities using a truck or van, facilities must consult the U.S. Department of Transportation, as well as state and local laws for transporting biohazardous items.
    *   *a.   True*   *(127)*

10. One goal of point-of-use preparation is to prevent instruments from being damaged.
    *   *a.   True*   *(120)*

1. What is the preferred pH for detergents used for most cleaning processes?
    c.   *Neutral pH*   *(147)*

2. Which of the following statements about the use of mechanical washers is NOT true?
    d.   *All items should be washed on the same cycle*   *(144)*

3. Water must be degassed each time the ultrasonic cleaner's tank is changed, because
    a.   *excess bubbles from filling reduce the energy of the cavitation process.*   *(140)*

4. Written cleaning instructions for surgical instruments should be provided by
    b.   *the device manufacturer.*   *(152)*

5. Pyrogens
    a.   *are fever-producing substances.*   *(135)*

6. Untreated water
    a.   *increases the likelihood of mineral scale deposits.*   *(136)*

7. These are used to breakdown fatty tissue on instruments.
    b.   *Lipase enzymes*   *(146)*

8. Instrument lubrication is performed
    c.   *after cleaning.*   *(149)*

9. To prevent coagulation of proteins, instruments should be pre-rinsed using
    a.   *cool water.*   *(142)*

10. Detergents used in mechanical cleaners should be
    d.   *low foaming.*   *(148)*

11. Instruments should be cleaned using a
    b.   *to and fro motion.*   *(153)*

12. Powered surgical instruments
    a.   *cannot be immersed.*   *(157)*

13. The decontamination area should have
    a.   *negative air flow in relation to the other areas of the department.*   *(132)*

14. The temperature in the decontamination area should be between
    c.   *60 to 65 degrees Fahrenheit.*   *(132)*

15. Rigid container filter retention plates should be
    a.   *removed from the container and lid and cleaned separately.*   *(151)*

Chapter 9: Disinfection Review Quiz   <u>*page reference*</u>

1. This low-level disinfectant is incompatible with soap.
    c.   Quaternary ammonium compounds   *(164)*

2. When using glutaraldehyde, technicians should always wear latex gloves for protection.
    b.   False   *(168)*

3. When using high-level disinfectants it is important to remember they may be deactivated by
    b.   organic matter.   *(167)*

4. In an automated washer the key source of disinfection is
    b.   water temperature.   *(173)*

5. The use of test strips to test the minimum effective concentration in high-level disinfection solutions is required
    c.   each time the solution will be used.   *(169)*

6. The use of heat to kill all microorganisms, except spores, is called
    b.   thermal disinfection.   *(173)*

7. These chemicals are used on animate (living tissue) to slow the growth of microorganisms.
    d.   Antiseptics   *(165)*

8. Items that are introduced directly into the bloodstream or other normally sterile areas of the body are classified as
    a.   critical items.   *(162)*

9. The process by which all forms of microorganisms are completely destroyed is called
    c.   sterilization.   *(163)*

10. Iodophors are a member of this chemical family.
    a.   Halogens   *(167)*

11. Phenolics are classified as
    a.   intermediate to low-level disinfectants.   *(165)*

12. Which of the following are classified as high-level disinfectants?
    b.   Glutaraldehyde and ortho-phthalaldehydes   *(168-169)*

13. Thermal disinfection is accomplished using
    d.   heat.   *(173)*

14. How long must alcohol remain in wet contact with an item to achieve a reasonable level of disinfection?
    c.   Five to 10 minutes   *(165)*

15. Which of the following would be the best choice for high-level disinfection of instruments?
    d.   Ortho-phthalaldehydes   *(169)*

1. Microgrind or supercut scissors are usually identified with a black handle.
   a. True   *(189)*

2. Stainless steel jaw needle holders last longer than tungsten carbide jaw needle holders.
   b. False   *(184)*

3. The place where the two parts of a ring handled instrument meet and pivot is called the box lock.
   a. True   *(183)*

4. Instruments are heat treated to give their surface a mirror (shiny) finish.
   b. False   *(182)*

5. Tissue forceps have teeth.
   a. True   *(186)*

6. During instrument manufacture the process of passivation helps build a protective chromium oxide layer on each instrument's surface.
   a. True   *(183)*

7. The part of a hemostat that locks and holds it in position is called the box lock.
   b. False   *(183)*

8. After applying instrument identification tape, instruments should be autoclaved to help the tape bond to the instrument.
   a. True   *(198)*

9. Instrument marking tape should be wrapped approximately _____ around the instrument.
   a. 1.5 times   *(198)*

10. An osteotome is
    a. used to cut or shave bone.   *(182)*

11. The purpose of a suction stylet is to
    a. unclog the suction during surgery.   *(191)*

12. Kerrison/laminectomy rongeurs should be tested using
    d. an index card.   *(196)*

13. Scissors with tungsten carbide cutting edges are usually identified by
    c. gold handles.   *(190)*

14. The best way to clean a suction lumen is
    b. using the proper sized brush.   *(191)*

15. To properly test the sharpness of scissors four inches or less use
    a. yellow test material.   *(196)*

1. The first step to inspect the insulation of a laparoscopic instrument is to
    a. *check the collar at the distal tip.*   *(217)*

2. Which of the following steps happens first when processing flexible endoscopes?
    a. *Leak-testing*   *(222)*

3. Which of the following should be used to thoroughly rinse (remove)
    all traces of disinfectant from an endoscope's channels?
    c. *Treated water*   *(225)*

4. The purpose of using a decontamination battery or hose when cleaning
    powered surgical instruments is
    a. *to keep fluid from entering the unit.*   *(207 & 209)*

5. Endoscopes are often processed in a mechanical unit called
    d. *an automatic endoscope reprocessor.*   *(227)*

6. The endoscope that would be dispensed for a procedure that required
    visualization of the lower part of the large intestine would be a
    b. *sigmoidoscope.*   *(221)*

7. Loaner instruments should
    c. *be decontaminated before use.*   *(240)*

8. Information regarding cleaning processes for endoscopes should be provided by
    c. *the instrument manufacturer.*   *(229)*

9. Which of the following statements about endoscopes is true?
    a. *Not all endoscopes can be processed in an automatic endoscope*
        reprocessor.   *(228)*

10. Electronic testing of laparoscopic insulation should be done
    b. *in the clean assembly area prior to set assembly.*   *(218)*

11. Loaner instrumentation can cause receiving challenges.
    a. *True*   *(239)*

12. Flexible endoscopes that fail a leak test may continue to be used until the
    break/hole impacts the scope's function.
    b. *False*   *(224)*

13. All flexible endoscopes have internal channels.
    b. *False*   *(221)*

14. After use, loaner instrumentation must be decontaminated before it is shipped out.
    a. *True*   *(241)*

15. The biggest advantage to battery-powered surgical instruments is that they can be
    immersed for cleaning.
    b. *False*   *(205)*

1. The U.S. Food and Drug Administration classifies sterilization packaging as a
    b.   Class II Medical Device   *(259)*

2. Which of the following is NOT an acceptable sterilization packaging material?
    c.   Canvas   *(260)*

3. Count sheets
    c.   provide a detailed list of tray contents.   *(247)*

4. When arranging paper/plastic pouches in the sterilizer, the pouches should be arranged
    a.   paper-to-plastic.   *(287)*

5. The relative humidity of the Central Service prep and pack area should be
    b.   30% to 60%.   *(244)*

6. Some plastics including formulations of spun-bonded polyolefin are intended for
    use solely in these sterilization processes
    b.   ozone and hydrogen peroxide.   *(266)*

7. When placing hinged instruments in an instrument tray, you should
    d.   unlock the handles and open the instruments.   *(255)*

8. Gauze squares are the wicking material of choice for instrument sets.
    b.   False   *(255)*

9. Temperatures in a sterile storage area should be 55°F to 60°F.
    b.   False   *(244)*

10. When placing instruments in a peel pack, the tips should always face the plastic
    side of the pack.
    a.   True   *(268)*

11. All rigid sterilization containers have tamper-evident seals.
    a.   True   *(284)*

12. Cellulose materials cannot be processed within ozone sterilizers.
    a.   True   *(259)*

13. Reusable textile packaging requires less labor than disposable packaging.
    b.   False   *(260)*

14. Using latex tubing to protect delicate instrumentation is the process of choice for items to
    be steam sterilized.
    b.   False   *(253)*

15. While the outside of all instruments must be dry before sterilization it is important to
    ensure all lumens are kept moist for sterilization.
    b.   False   *(248)*

1. The process by which instruments are steam sterilized for immediate use is called
   b.   *immediate use steam sterilization.*   *(292)*

2. Items to be disinfected or sterilized at the point of use must be
   a.   *properly cleaned per manufacturer's Instructions for Use.*   *(292 & 296)*

3. The best way to transport items that have been processed using immediate use steam sterilization at the point of use is
   b.   *in a rigid container designed for immediate use steam sterilization.*   *(296)*

4. Before an item can be placed in a liquid chemical sterile processing system they must be
   d.   *cleaned.*   *(295)*

5. Which of the following statements about immediate use steam sterilization is true?
   d.   *It should be used only when there is not time to process items using the wrapped method*   *(292)*

6. Both the Association of periOperative Registered Nurses and The Joint Commission recommend that
   a.   *the use of immediate use steam sterilization be minimized or decreased.*   *(293-94)*

7. Implantable devices
   c.   *should not be immediate use steam sterilization sterilized unless there is a tracking system in place to trace the item to a patient.*   *(294)*

8. When transporting items that have been immediate use steam sterilized, it is required that
   d.   *they be transported in such a manner that reduces the potential for contamination.*   *(296)*

9. When sterilizing items at the point of use, an abbreviated sterilization cycle may be used due to the urgent need for the instruments.
   b.   *False*   *(295)*

10. Immediate use steam sterilization documentation should include
    d.   *all the above.*   *(297)*

Chapter 14: High-Temperature Sterilization Review Quiz   <u>*page reference*</u>

1. When loading a steam sterilizer, basins should be
   c.   *placed on edge.*   *(315)*

2. The higher the bioburden on an object
   a.   *the more difficult it will be to sterilize.*   *(302)*

3. When combining loads, hard goods should be placed on the top shelves to allow for more efficient removal of the condensate.
   b.   *False*

4. The steam sterilization process can be affected by the design of the medical device being sterilized.
    a. True   (302)

5. Central Service technicians need to understand the anatomy of a steam sterilizer to
    b. understand how the sterilizer operates.   (303)

6. The weakest part of a steam sterilizer is the
    c. door.   (305)

7. Three of the main phases of a terminal steam sterilizer cycle are
    d. conditioning, exposure and exhaust.   (308)

8. The most common reason for steam sterilization failure is
    a. lack of steam contact with the instrument.   (311)

9. The coolest place in a steam sterilizer is the
    b. thermostatic valve.   (306)

10. Steam flush pressure pulse sterilizers are a type of gravity sterilizers.
    b. False   (307)

11. Factors that can cause sterilant contact failure with the instrument are
    d. crowded loads, clogged drain strainer.   (311-12)

12. One of the most frequent causes of a clogged drain screen is
    a. tape.   (312)

13. After sterilization the load contents may take two hours or more to cool.
    a. True   (316)

14. Peel pouches should be placed _____ for sterilization.
    a. on edge, paper to plastic   (316)

15. Items with a standard steam sterilization cycle recommended by the manufacturer can be damaged if run in an extended cycle.
    a. True   (319)

16. How frequently should a sterilizer's strainer be removed and cleaned?
    a. Daily   (305)

17. Immediate use steam sterilization is the process to sterilize trays for future use.
    b. False   (308)

18. Wood products should be sterilized in an extended steam cycle.
    b. False   (315)

19. When water is seen on the outside of a pack after sterilization the pack is considered safe to use if all other packs in the load are dry.
    b. False   (317)

20. Packs that are improperly packaged or loaded on the sterilizer cart frequently become wet packs.
    a. True   (318)

Chapter 15: Low-Temperature Sterilization Review Quiz   <u>*page reference*</u>

1. Woven reusable fabrics are the packaging products of choice for ozone sterilization.
   b. *False*   *(336)*

2. Ethylene kills microorganisms by a process called oxidation.
   b. *False*   *(323)*

3. Ethylene oxide, hydrogen peroxide and ozone sterilization process must all be monitored using chemical, physical and biological monitors.
   a. *True*   *(322)*

4. Ethylene oxide, hydrogen peroxide and ozone sterilization can all use the same packaging materials.
   b. *False*   *(327, 331, 336)*

5. Lumens should be moist when using hydrogen peroxide as a sterilizing agent.
   b. *False*   *(331)*

6. Ethylene oxide is a toxic gas.
   a. *True*   *(325)*

7. Cellulose-containing packaging materials are not compatible with hydrogen peroxide sterilization.
   a. *True*   *(331)*

8. Information about a device's compatibility with a specific sterilization process should be obtained from the device's manufacturer.
   a. *True*   *(326)*

9. An extended aeration cycle is required for items sterilized in ozone sterilization processes.
   b. *False*   *(337)*

10. Permissible exposure levels for low-temperature sterilization methods are established by the
    c. *Occupational Safety and Health Administration.*   *(323)*

1. The relative humidity of the Central Service sterile storage area should be
   - a. *less than 70%.*   *(344)*

2. Temperatures in a sterile storage area should be 64^0 to 75^0 F.
   - b. *False*   *(344)*

3. Because of event-related shelf life, stock rotation is no longer necessary.
   - b. *False*   *(352)*

4. The sterile storage process starts
   - c. *when the sterilizer door is opened.*   *(342)*

5. Sterile storage areas should
   - b. *have positive airflow and at least four air exchanges per hour.*   *(344)*

6. Temperature and humidity levels in the sterile storage area should be checked and recorded at least weekly.
   - b. *False*   *(344)*

7. The shelving system of choice for the sterile storage area is
   - a. *closed.*   *(345)*

8. Trays which overhang shelving
   - a. *can become contaminated.*   *(344)*

9. The type of shelving that leaves packaging the most vulnerable is
   - a. *open.*   *(346)*

10. The bottom shelf of any sterile storage system should be
    - a. *solid and eight to 10 inches from the floor.*   *(346)*

11. Sterile trays should
    - d. *all the above.*   *(347)*

12. Wrapped trays should not be stacked because
    - b. *it can cause holes in the wrapper of the bottom tray.*   *(347)*

13. Outside shipping containers
    - a. *should be removed prior to placing the items in storage.*   *(348)*

14. Event-related shelf life means items are safe until opened for use.
    - b. *False*   *(349)*

15. Sterilized packages may be jeopardized due to storage practices.
    - a. *True*   *(349)*

Chapter 17: Monitoring and Recordkeeping for Central Service Review Quiz

page reference

1. Formal training should occur
   - d. *for new employees and those who move to new positions.*   *(371)*

2. Monitoring records must be
   - d. *all the above.*   *(358)*

3. Sterilizer load records should contain
   - a. *items and quantity sterilized.*   *(366)*

4. External indicators can prove an item is sterile when the sterilization cycle is complete.
   - b. *False*   *(362)*

5. Temperature and humidity levels need to be monitored and recorded
   - c. *at least daily.*   *(359)*

6. The FDA Class II chemical indicator that is run daily in dynamic air removal sterilizers is called a
   - d. *Bowie-Dick test.*   *(369)*

7. One type of formal monitoring is monitoring the department temperature and humidity levels.
   - a. *True*   *(359)*

8. A physical monitor on a washer-disinfector is the
   - b. *printout.*   *(361)*

9. Cart washer screens should be cleaned at least
   - a. *daily.*   *(361)*

10. A biological indicator is called positive when
    - b. *there is no growth in the ampule after incubation.*   *(364)*

Chapter 18: Quality Assurance Review Quiz

page reference

1. Quality requires the efforts and participation of everyone in the healthcare facility.
   - a. *True*   *(374)*

2. A failure mode and effects analysis tries to predict failures before they occur.
   - a. *True*   *(379-80)*

3. The International Standards Organization uses routine and unannounced inspections to monitor standards in healthcare facilities.
   - b. *False*   *(386)*

4. Quality processes are limited to administration and the risk management department.
   - b. *False*   *(375)*

171

5. Quality management is patient focused.
   a. True (377)

6. Providing quality products and services directly impacts patient outcomes.
   b. False (374)

7. Customer surveys are ineffective tools in establishing Central Service quality processes.
   b. False (375)

8. If everyone develops a quality-driven focus, written policies and procedures are not necessary in the Central Service department.
   b. False (386)

9. A root cause analysis is a proactive approach to quality.
   b. False (380)

10. Not following established policies and procedures will result in a lower quality program.
    a. True (386)

Chapter 19: Managing Inventory within the Central Service Department
Review Quiz   *page reference*

1. Which of the following systems provides supplies and instruments for individual surgical procedures?
   c. Case cart (401)

2. The inventory system that stocks supplies by established stock levels is called
   a. a periodic automated replenishment system (399)

3. The inventory system that uses two identical carts to facilitate supply replenishment is called the
   b. exchange cart system. (400)

4. Automated supply replenishment systems are
   d. computerized. (399)

5. The movement of supplies throughout the healthcare facility is called
   a. distribution. (398)

6. Operational supplies are supplies that are dispensed for patient care.
   b. False (393)

7. Supplies such as disposable wraps are called
   a. consumable. (393)

8. Capital equipment items are
   c. items with a higher purchase cost. (393)

9. The following symbolizes

    d.   *product manufacture date.*   *(396)*

10. The following symbolizes

    b.   *use by date.*   *(396)*

Chapter 20: The Role of Central Service in Ancillary Department Support
Review Quiz   *page reference*

1. Technicians in the _____ department perform safety inspections and functional tests on equipment.
      c.   *Biomedical engineering*   *(410)*

2. When patient equipment enters a healthcare facility, it must be safety checked by a _____ before it is cleared for patient use.
      a.   *Biomedical technician*   *(410)*

3. Which of the following requires that preventive maintenance standards be established for medical equipment?
      b.   *The Joint Commission*   *(410)*

4. All patient care equipment that was dispensed for use must be considered _____, and handled as such, regardless of its appearance.
      c.   *contaminated*   *(411)*

5. Which of the following common items of patient care equipment limits the development of deep vein thrombosis and peripheral edema in immobile patients?
      c.   *Sequential compression unit*   *(409)*

6. Disposable components such as pads and tubing on patient care equipment should be
      a.   *discarded at the point of use.*   *(411)*

7. Equipment should be inspected for obvious hazards such as cracked or frayed electrical cords
      d.   *whenever the equipment is inspected in Central Service.*   *(411)*

8. If an equipment malfunction causes harm to patients, it should be
      d.   *returned immediately to the biomedical department.*   *(411)*

9. Patient care equipment should be stored in a _____ condition.
    a.   *"ready to dispense"*   *(412)*

10. Patient care equipment is typically stored
    c.   *in the Central Service department.*   *(412)*

11. The _____ requires that the healthcare facility report malfunctions of medical devices that have contributed to patient injury, illness and/or death to the manufacturer and the U.S. Food and Drug Administration.
    b.   *Safe Medical Devices Act*   *(412)*

12. Which of the following statements is correct?
    c.   *Tracking patient care equipment can prevent equipment shortages*   *(413)*

13. Equipment leasing and rental differ in that
    b.   *equipment rental is usually done on a shorter-term basis than equipment leasing.*   *(412)*

14. Preventive maintenance is
    b.   *designed to identify potential problems before they occur.*   *(410)*

15. The decision to use reusable or disposable instruments in procedure trays is determined by
    c.   *several factors including physician preference, storage and cost.*   *(415)*

Chapter 21: The Role of Information Technology in Central Service
Review Quiz   *page reference*

1. In addition to providing financial and operational management, information technology and systems are used to help ensure patient safety.
    a.   *True*   *(419)*

2. Information technology is often the cornerstone of initiatives to transform healthcare.
    a.   *True*   *(419)*

3. Which of the following is NOT a result of computer integration?
    c.   *Automatically provides critical update to industry standards*   *(419)*

4. Patient census information used in Central Service is obtained from the electronic health record.
    b.   *False*   *(420)*

5. Computer supply chain management systems are used to monitor facility assets.
    b.   *False*   *(421)*

6. Tracking individual instruments is important to help ensure specific instruments are kept with a specific set.
    a.   *True*   *(425)*

7. Which of the following is NOT a reason for tracking supplies, equipment and instruments?
    *c. Meeting Centers for Disease Control and Occupational Safety and Health
       Administration requirements* (418)

8. Which of the following tracking methods provides real-time information?
    a. Radio frequency identification tags (423)

9. Point-of-use computing
    c. moves computers into Central Service work areas. (419)

10. Which of the following is NOT a feature of an instrument tracking system?
    d. Product updates and recall information (426)

11. Computerized tracking systems are fast, but manual tracking systems are more
    effective for tracking.
    b. False (424)

12. Once a tracking system is implemented, there is generally no need to update system
    information.
    b. False (424)

13. At this time, tracking systems are unable to track worker productivity information.
    b. False (426)

14. Tracking systems can help manage preventive maintenance schedules.
    a. True (426)

15. Most Central Service departments employ some sort of automated information
    management system.
    a. True (418)

Chapter 22: Safety and Risk Management for Central Service Review Quiz <u>*page reference*</u>

1. Risk management programs are designed to prevent accidents and injury.
    a. True (430)

2. Which of the following is NOT a component of risk management?
    c. Staff management (430)

3. Which of the following is NOT considered one of the three types of occupational hazards?
    b. Ergonomic hazards (431-32)

4. Information about chemical or hazardous substances must be available to all employees.
    a. True (435)

5. Healthcare facilities are required by the _____ to provide adequate
    ventilation systems, personal protective equipment and safe work operating procedures?
    c. Occupational Safety and Health Administration (437)

6. Time-weighted average is defined as the amount of a substance you can be exposed to over an eight-hour day.
    a. *True* (442)

7. The process of changing work or working conditions to reduce physical stress is
    a. *called ergonomics.* (432)

8. The key to working safely is keeping your work area organized.
    b. *False* (431)

9. When you cannot see what is in a sink or basin you should
    b. *use a sponge forceps to grasp items.* (439)

10. Which of the following is NOT required for sharps safety?
    c. *Wash all disposable sharps before discarding them* (434)

11. The level of exposure to a harmful substance when an employer must take required precautions to protect the worker.
    d. *Action level* (442)

12. Ergonomic injuries
    c. *are a risk factor for persons who perform repetitive or physical work.* (431)

13. Secondary containers of chemicals
    a. *must be labeled with a copy of the original manufacturer's label or a generic label that identifies hazard warnings and directions.* (436)

14. Safety data sheets are provided by the
    d. *product manufacturer.* (436)

15. A molecular reaction that creates an uncontrolled release of energy is called
    b. *polymerization.* (436)

Chapter 23: Success through Communication Review Quiz   *page reference*

1. Which of the following is an example of communication?
    d. *All of the above* (452)

2. Central Service technicians who do not think they are being treated appropriately by their employer should
    c. *discuss the situation with their supervisor.* (454)

3. Behavior relating to what is "right and wrong" relative to the standards of conduct for your profession are called
    a. *ethical behavior.* (455)

4. A step in communication that occurs when a listener asks a question is called
    b. *feedback.* (455)

5. This process allows a person to understand someone else's needs.
    a. *Communication*   *(452)*

6. When speaking, you should
    b. *concentrate on the listener rather than oneself.*   *(456)*

7. Which of the following basic listening tactics is most useful?
    d. *None of the above*   *(456)*

8. The ability to use information gained from words or body language to
    interact with others.
    a. *Communication*   *(452)*

9. Which of the following is the most important factor necessary for teamwork?
    a. *Attitude*   *(460)*

10. Which of the following statements is correct?
    b. *Informal work groups develop an informal communication system called the
    grapevine*   *(462)*

11. A group of employees from different departments within the healthcare facility
    that work together to solve operating problems is called a
    c. *cross-functional team.*   *(462)*

12. Which of the following is true about a valuing diversity effort?
    d. *None of the above*   *(463)*

13. Coaching is an example of
    c. *formal communication.*   *(457)*

14. Knowing what is expected and consistently meeting those expectations is part of
    d. *professional behavior.*   *(454)*

15. When Central Service technicians have internet access at work
    d. *they should follow the facility's policy.*   *(458)*

1. Which of the following is an open-ended question?
    c. *"What problems do you most frequently encounter on the job?"*   *(473)*

2. Personal development improves your employability skills.
    a. *True*   *(468)*

3. When setting personal goals you should set goals that are
    c. *attainable, then build on those successes.*   *(468)*

4. Professional development helps give you the information and experience needed to progress in your career.
    a. *True*   *(468)*

5. Teaching others increases your understanding of the standards.
    a. *True*   *(470)*

6. Planning and reviewing your goals will help identify activities to help you meet those goals.
    a. *True*   *(470)*

7. Resources found online have already been determined to be valid before they are posted online.
    b. *False*   *(471)*

8. Steps toward attaining professional goals in Central Service include
    d. *all the above.*   *(471)*

9. One important step in preparing for an interview is
    c. *anticipating possible interview questions.*   *(473)*

10. On the job relationships do NOT change when one team member has been promoted.
    b. *False*   *(474)*

PROGRESS TEST ONE

Complete the following 20 multiple choice and true/false questions.

1. A pick list contains information that
   a. assists the surgeon during the procedure.
   b. is used to assemble surgery instrument sets.
   c. assists the Central Service technician in selecting the correct supplies for the sterile storage area.
   d. identifies the supplies and instruments needed for a specific doctor and procedure.

2. The basic unit of a living organism.
   a. Cell
   b. Cytoplasm
   c. Nucleus
   d. Organ

3. What is the name of the surgical procedure where an opening is made into the skull?
   a. Burr holes
   b. Craniotomy
   c. Craniectomy
   d. Open reduction of the skull

4. The decontamination area of the Central Service department is where instruments are carefully checked for cleanliness and function.
   a. True
   b. False

5. The term "periosteal elevator" means
   a. surgical removal of tissue near the thyroid.
   b. surgical removal of one half of the stomach.
   c. an instrument for cutting skin.
   d. an instrument used to remove tissue around the bone.

6. Viruses
   a. move by a droplet method of transportation.
   b. move by a direct contact method of transportation.
   c. move by an airborne method of transportation.
   d. have no means of movement on their own.

7. The sterile storage area in a Central Service department should be restricted to
   a. Central Service managers and supervisors.
   b. Operating Room personnel.
   c. Central Service employees only.
   d. properly attired personnel meeting facility requirements.

8. The abbreviation *BKA* refers to a surgical procedure involving
    a. treatment of a fractured bone without a surgical incision.
    b. surgical removal of both the fallopian tubes and ovaries.
    c. surgical removal of the leg below the knee.
    d. a type of hip joint reconstruction.

9. The body's control center is the
    a. meninges.
    b. central nervous system.
    c. the brain stem.
    d. cerebrum.

10. The prefix word element
    a. comes immediately before the suffix.
    b. comes before the root.
    c. comes before the suffix and describes the word meaning.
    d. comes after the suffix.

11. The muscular system
    a. assists with movement.
    b. produces heat for the body.
    c. pumps blood throughout the body.
    d. is all of the above.

12. Microbes
    a. can be useful in food products.
    b. are useful to break down sewage.
    c. can produce toxins.
    d. are all of the above.

13. Prefix, suffix and roots are called word elements and are contained in all medical terms.
    a. True
    b. False

14. The pupil of the eye is the
    a. middle layer of the eye.
    b. colored portion of the eye.
    c. white portion of the eye.
    d. circular opening that controls the amount of light entering the eye.

15. Skin is a type of connective tissue.
    a. True
    b. False

16. An advantage of centralizing Central Service management is
    a. payroll costs are lower.
    b. more instruments can be processed faster than in a decentralized department.
    c. allows for maximization of people and services.
    d. there are no real advantages to centralization.

17. Prions are
    a. abnormal forms of protein.
    b. gram positive bacillus.
    c. a type of virus.
    d. an acid fast microorganism.

18. A herniorrhaphy is a surgical procedure which
    a. repairs a shoulder muscle.
    b. repairs a muscle layer that is allowing all or part of an organ to project through an opening.
    c. removes a sample of diseased or infected muscle.
    d. repairs fibrous membranes that cover a muscle.

19. The abbreviation *CR* relates to a surgical procedure for
    a. treating a fractured bone without a surgical incision.
    b. creating a new blood supply to an area of the heart.
    c. surgical removal of the uterus.
    d. surgical removal of part of the prostate gland.

20. Bacteria which cause disease are called
    a. gram positive.
    b. gram negative.
    c. pathogens.
    d. potentially infectious.

PROGRESS TEST TWO

Complete the following 40 multiple choice and true/false questions.

1. The U.S. Food and Drug Administration is responsible for
   a. maintaining all manufacturer records.
   b. ensuring items can be properly cleaned and sterilized.
   c. monitoring the high-level disinfection process.
   d. ensuring food, drugs and cosmetics are safe for use.

2. The basics of aseptic technique is
   a. knowing the chain of infection.
   b. activities that prevent infection.
   c. following the Bloodborne Pathogen Standard.
   d. all the above.

3. The decontamination area of the Central Service department should have
   a. negative air flow.
   b. positive air flow.
   c. filtered air flow.
   d. no air exchanges because it is a biohazard area.

4. Decontamination of instruments and equipment starts
   a. during the manual cleaning process.
   b. as soon as the instruments are received in the decontamination area.
   c. at the point of use.
   d. when the instruments are placed back in their trays at the point of use.

5. The decontamination area should have
   a. negative air flow in relation to the other areas of the department.
   b. positive air flow in relation to the other areas of the department.
   c. 15 air exchanges per hour.
   d. positive air flow with 15 exchanges per hour.

6. The proper handling of instrumentation is the responsibility of
   a. the surgeon.
   b. the scrub technician.
   c. the Central Service technician.
   d. everyone who comes in contact with the instrumentation.

7. Centers for Disease Control guidelines are considered regulatory guidelines.
   a. True
   b. False

8. One of the goals of point-of-use preparation and transport is to
   a. speed up the decontamination process.
   b. ensure all the instruments are returned to Central Service.
   c. prevent cross contamination.
   d. all the above.

9. Automatic washers clean using a spray-force action called impingement.
    a. True
    b. False

10. The federal program designed for the voluntary reporting of device related problems is called
    a. the Safe Medical Device Act.
    b. the Medical Device Recall Act
    c. the U.S. Food and Drug Administration reporting requirements.
    d. MedWatch.

11. When removing personal protective equipment you should remove _____ first.
    a. gloves
    b. gown
    c. mask
    d. shoe covers

12. Which of the following tells a primary meaning of a word?
    a. Prefix word element
    b. Root word element
    c. Suffix word element
    d. Combining vowel

13. In Central Service, the concept of "one-way flow of materials" refers to the movement of products
    a. from Central Service to surgical areas.
    b. from surgical areas to Central Service.
    c. from soiled areas to clean processing areas within Central Service.
    d. from clean processing areas to soiled areas in Central Service.

14. Which of these traffic control/dress code requirements applies to the clean assembly area of Central Service?
    a. Biohazard
    b. Unrestricted
    c. Semi restricted
    d. Restricted

15. End of procedure point-of-use guideline include removing gross soil, disassembling of multi-part instruments, and ensuring instruments are kept moist.
    a. True
    b. False

16. The Association of periOperative Registered Nurses is
    a. a regulatory agency that writes regulatory standards for the Operating Room.
    b. responsible for writing Infection Prevention guidelines.
    c. a voluntary agency that oversees professional standards.
    d. a professional organization that writes guidelines for the Operating Room.

17. When putting on personal protective equipment it is important to put the mask on first.
    a. True
    b. False

18. To prevent aerosols, items should be brushed below the surface of the water.
    a. True
    b. False

19. The suffix -*ectomy* means
    a. to repair
    b. surgical removal
    c. inflammation
    d. None of the above

20. This surgical procedure removes the uterus.
    a. Hysteroscopy
    b. Hysterectomy
    c. Dilatation & curettage
    d. Bilateral-salpingo oophorectomy

21. When cleaning prion contaminated instruments no special cleaning procedures are required only following standard cleaning protocols and the Manufacturer's Instructions for Use.
    a. True
    b. False

22. Healthy people do not harbor or transmit bacteria.
    a. True
    b. False

23. When cleaning items contaminated with pseudomonas
    a. items should be cleaned in a separate area to prevent cross-contamination.
    b. items should be placed in a disinfectant solution prior to manual cleaning.
    c. the Infection Prevention department should be notified of the contamination.
    d. there are no special cleaning requirements for items contaminated with pseudomonas.

24. The purpose of learning medical terminology is
    a. to give the central service technician an understanding of Latin and French words.
    b. to enable central service technicians to read instrument count sheets.
    c. to provide the Operating Room and medical staff with the goods and services they need.
    d. to list critical terms used in the healthcare setting.

25. Which organization conducts onsite survey of healthcare facilities?
    a. Society of Gastroenterology Nurses and Associates
    b. Association for Professionals in Infection Control and Epidemiology
    c. American National Standards Institute
    d. The Joint Commission

26. All Central Service departments perform the same basic services.
    a. True
    b. False

27. Knowing and understanding medical terminology helps technicians
    a. reduce the productivity of the Operating Room.
    b. understand manufacturer's Instructions for Use.
    c. understand what is asked when a request is made.
    d. become proficient in Latin and French word elements.

28. *Hypoglycemia* means
    a. a malignant tumor.
    b. tissue death of an artery.
    c. low blood sugar.
    d. enlargement of the heart.

29. If soiled instruments are to be transported to an offsite facility for processing
    a. they should be counted prior to placing them in the transport vehicle.
    b. they should be placed in special containers made for instrument transport.
    c. they should be transported following the U.S. or state Department of Transportation guidelines.
    d. they should be transported following the Association for Professionals in Infection Control and Epidemiology safe transportation guidelines.

30. All mechanical cleaning equipment provides
    a. multiple cleaning cycles.
    b. pre-rinse, wash, rinse, lubrication and dry cycles.
    c. consistent process.
    d. all the above.

31. Microbiology is the study of
    a. life.
    b. microorganisms.
    c. human immune systems.
    d. all the above.

32. Detergents used in mechanical cleaners should be
    a. low alkaline.
    b. low acid.
    c. low temperature.
    d. low foaming.

33. Which of the following is NOT a growing trend in Central Service?
    a. Decentralization of Central Service responsibilities
    b. The use of more reusable and more complex devices
    c. Satellite-processing units with centralized management
    d. Consolidation into entire integrated delivery networks

34. Subcutaneous means
    a. low sugar content in the blood.
    b. displacement of the pelvic joint.
    c. beneath the skin.
    d. without infection; sterile.

35. Spores help some microorganisms survive in adverse conditions.
    a. True
    b. False

36. Which of the following surgical abbreviations might be used relating to a fractured bone?
    a. CABG
    b. BSO
    c. ORIF
    d. TAH

37. Only good oral and written communication skills are necessary to provide or obtain information.
    a. True
    b. False

38. Soiled instruments and other items are received in the _____ area of the Central service department.
    a. preparation
    b. packaging
    c. decontamination
    d. sterilization

39. A system is
    a. a group of organs.
    b. two or more different types of tissue.
    c. a group of living cells that join together.
    d. all the above.

40. The procedure to remove the stomach
    a. gastritis.
    b. gastrectomy.
    c. gastric bypass.
    d. gastric sleeve.

PROGRESS TEST THREE

Complete the following 60 multiple choice and true/false questions.

1. The system used to categorize patient care items based on the degree of risk of infection.
   a. Ziehl-Neelsen Classification System
   b. Medical Device Classification System
   c. Spaulding Classification System
   d. High-level Disinfection Classification System

2. An osteotome is
   a. used to cut or shave bone.
   b. a retractor.
   c. a hemostatic forceps.
   d. none of the above.

3. When returning loaner items to the vendor
   a. all items should be completely assembled, tested and sterile.
   b. trays should be returned immediately after point-of-use cleaning.
   c. all items should be cleaned and decontaminated.
   d. trays should be terminally sterilized before returning them to the vendor.

4. The first goal of creating an instrument pack is
   a. obtain the proper packaging container for the pack.
   b. decide on the order of instrument placement.
   c. create a pack that meets user needs.
   d. create a pack that makes the physician happy.

5. Positive air flow means when the door is opened, air flows out of instead of into the area.
   a. True
   b. False

6. Molds, mushrooms and yeast are common
   a. gram-negative organisms.
   b. fungi.
   c. gram-positive organisms.
   d. prions.

7. The surgery of the ear that reconstructs the eardrum so sound waves can be sent to the middle ear
   a. tympanoplasty.
   b. stapedectomy.
   c. auditory implantation.
   d. myringotomy.

8. Dark areas on the lens of an endoscope are?
   a. Debris
   b. Light-emitting diode optics
   c. Light-emitting diode bulbs
   d. Damaged light fibers

9. Soiled instruments and other items are received in the _____ area of the Central Service department.
   a. preparation
   b. packaging
   c. decontamination
   d. sterilization

10. Pasteurizers disinfect using
    a. heated water.
    b. phenols.
    c. high-level disinfectants.
    d. peracetic acid.

11. Which of the following statements about the use of mechanical washers is NOT true?
    a. Multi-level trays should be separated
    b. Trays with lids should be opened
    c. Instruments should be disassembled and opened
    d. All items should be washed on the same cycle

12. Agency which may intervene in a matter of worker protection even if there are no specific regulations covering the situation.
    a. Occupational Safety and Health Administration
    b. Environmental Protection Agency
    c. U.S. Food and Drug Administration
    d. Association of periOperative Registered Nurses

13. Laser finished instruments are coated with a durable protective finish that cannot be chipped or scratched.
    a. True
    b. False

14. Healthcare-associated infections are
    a. most likely to occur during a surgical procedure.
    b. caused by drug resistant organisms.
    c. those without known cures.
    d. those which occur in the course of being treated in a healthcare facility.

15. Viruses are larger than bacteria.
    a. True
    b. False

16. The system that gives the body shape and support
    a. muscular system.
    b. nervous system.
    c. skeletal system.
    d. circulatory system.

17. Devices categorized as semi-critical items, must be at least _____ prior to use.
    a. high-level disinfected
    b. intermediate-level disinfected
    c. low-level disinfected
    d. sterilized

18. Electronic testing of laparoscopic insulation should be done
    a. in the decontamination area prior to cleaning.
    b. in the clean assembly area prior to set assembly.
    c. at the factory or onsite repair unit.
    d. in the operating room at the end of the procedure.

19. Count sheets
    a. describe each instrument in detail.
    b. are used only for Operating Room trays and large procedure packs.
    c. provide a detailed list of tray contents.
    d. all the above.

20. Central Service technicians must wear special attire referred to as _____ to minimize their exposure to bloodborne pathogens and other contaminants.
    a. PPE
    b. OSHA
    c. TPA
    d. CDC

21. The temperature in the decontamination area should be between
    a. 55 to 60 degrees Fahrenheit
    b. 58 to 62 degrees Fahrenheit
    c. 60 to 65 degrees Fahrenheit
    d. 65 to 70 degrees Fahrenheit

22. Staphylococcus is classified as a gram-positive bacteria.
    a. True
    b. False

23. Kerrison/laminectomy rongeurs should be tested using
    a. tissue paper.
    b. a plastic dowel rod.
    c. rubber testing material.
    d. an index card.

24. Which of the following should be used to thoroughly rinse (remove) all traces of disinfectant from an endoscope's channels?
    a. Forced air
    b. Water containing approved sterilant
    c. Treated water
    d. A heated glutaraldehyde

25. The prefix *hemi-*
    a. means near.
    b. is a suffix.
    c. means half.
    d. means around.

26. The term *septorhinoplasty* means
    a. surgery of a muscle wound.
    b. surgical repair of the nose.
    c. removal of a cyst.
    d. incision of the stomach.

27. Powered surgical instrument air hoses should be pressurized for proper inspection.
    a. True
    b. False

28. The use of test strips to test the minimum effective concentration in high-level disinfection solutions is required
    a. weekly preferably daily.
    b. Daily.
    c. each time the solution will be used.
    d. only when manual soaking systems are used.

29. Arthroscopy instruments are used during
    a. robotic surgery.
    b. laparoscopic surgery.
    c. joint surgery.
    d. all the above.

30. The term *itis* means
    a. illness.
    b. inflammation.
    c. study of.
    d. pain.

31. Bacteria that do not require free oxygen to live are called
    a. pathogenic.
    b. anaerobic.
    c. aerobic.
    d. vibrio.

32. Instruments with tungsten carbide jaws can be easily identified by
    a. the diamond serration pattern on the instrument jaws.
    b. the black handles on the instrument.
    c. the gold handles on the instrument.
    d. the self-retaining lock on the instrument shaft.

33. Robotic instruments
    a. do not come apart for cleaning.
    b. have mechanical and electrical components in the proximal end of the instrument.
    c. are heavier than standard laparoscopic instruments.
    d. are all of the above.

34. An important reason for instrument preparation to begin at the point of use is
    a. it decreases the turnaround times in Central Service.
    b. it helps prolong the life of the instruments.
    c. it reduces the amount of biohazardous waste being transported.
    d. it ensures all instruments are returned to Central Service.

35. The mechanical process by which an ultrasonic cleaner works is called cavitation.
    a. True
    b. False

36. Clean multi-part instruments that have been assembled to test for functionality should
    a. remain assembled for sterilization.
    b. be disassembled and placed in peel packs for sterilization.
    c. be disassembled and sterilized following manufacturer's Instructions for Use.
    d. broken down and placed in separate containers for sterilization.

37. To protect themselves from splashes and spills, Central Service technicians assigned to the decontamination area should wear
    a. double-cloth gowns.
    b. blue surgical scrubs.
    c. fluid-resistant gowns.
    d. sterile operating room gowns.

38. These are used to breakdown fatty tissue on instruments
    a. protease enzymes.
    b. lipase enzymes.
    c. amylase enzymes.
    d. neutral pH cleaners.

39. This is the lining of the uterus.
    a. Vagina
    b. Endometrium
    c. Fimbriae
    d. Skin

40. Healthcare regulations and standards provide consistency of departmental activities by outlining
    a. minimal levels of quality and safety.
    b. equal pay practices.
    c. productivity time lines.
    d. all of the above.

41. When a soiled instrument is found during the assembly process
    a. the instrument should be cleaned with a soft bristled brush and alcohol.
    b. the instrument should be discarded.
    c. the entire work area must be cleaned.
    d. the instrument and the tray it was in should be sent to the decontamination area for re-cleaning.

42. Skeletal muscles
    a. move involuntarily.
    b. move only when we want them to move.
    c. are responsible for muscle movement.
    d. all the above.

43. The virus that causes hepatitis B is transmitted by
    a. contact.
    b. blood.
    c. airborne.
    d. vector-borne.

44. Departmental dress codes apply to
    a. everyone entering the Central Service department.
    b. only hospital employees.
    c. only persons who will be spending more than 10 minutes in the Central Service work area.
    d. only visitors such as sales reps, maintenance personnel, etc.

45. All sonic cleaners have a decontamination cycle.
    a. True
    b. False

46. Chemical indicators are _____ devices.
    a. FDA Class I
    b. FDA Class II
    c. FDA Class III
    d. unregulated

47. The main theory of standard precautions is
    a. that patients in high-risk categories may be infectious.
    b. that patients diagnosed with a specific disease may be infectious.
    c. that patients are generally healthy unless they show symptoms of an infectious disease.
    d. to treat all human blood and body fluids as infectious.

48. Failure to perform soiled pick up rounds as scheduled can lead to instrument and equipment shortages.
    a. True
    b. False

49. Rigid container filter retention plates should be
    a. removed from the container and lid and cleaned separately.
    b. manually cleaned and attached to the lid for mechanical cleaning.
    c. left attached to the lid during the cleaning process.
    d. none of the above.

50. The absence of microorganisms that cause disease is called
    a. infection prevention.
    b. infection control.
    c. asepsis.
    d. healthcare-associated infection control.

51. The amount of time an item must remain wet with a disinfectant to achieve disinfection is called
    a. holding time.
    b. wet contact time.
    c. activation.
    d. sterilization time.

52. When an instrument has a shiny surface it is said to have a _____ finish.
    a. satin
    b. passivation
    c. matte
    d. mirror

53. The word *laminectomy* means
    a. removal of a cyst in the spine.
    b. removal of part of a lamina.
    c. to cut out part of a small bone.
    d. the study of the spine.

54. Recommendations regarding sterilization practices are provided by the Association for the Advancement of Medical Instrumentation.
    a. True
    b. False

55. Hand hygiene is considered the single most important factor in reducing infections.
    a. True
    b. False

56. Contaminated items may be returned to Central Service
    a. during scheduled soiled pick up rounds.
    b. by staff from user departments.
    c. in case carts.
    d. all the above.

57. Sometimes state or local regulations differ from federal regulations and when that happens, the most stringent regulations apply.
    a. True
    b. False

58. Items should be contained for transport
    a. to keep the instruments from unnecessary movement during transport.
    b. to keep the instrument sets intact.
    c. to minimize the spread of microorganisms.
    d. all the above.

59. Cleaning brushes
    a. should be cleaned and sterilized at least every daily.
    b. should have metal bristles.
    c. larger than the lumen to be cleaned.
    d. all the above.

60. The term *hypo* means
    a. quickly.
    b. above.
    c. below.
    d. measured.

PROGRESS TEST FOUR

Complete the following 100 multiple choice and true/false questions.

1. The process by which instruments are sterilized for immediate use is called
   a. emergency sterilization.
   b. Immediate Use Steam Sterilization.
   c. core sterilization.
   d. rapid reprocessing.

2. Steam sterilization is the most commonly used method of sterilization used in healthcare because
   a. cycles are fast and inexpensive.
   b. it is versatile; the temperature can be adjusted to sterilize heat sensitive items.
   c. there is no need to run biological tests for steam sterilization.
   d. chemical indicators are optional in steam sterilization.

3. When placing sterile items on the shelf you should check
   a. package integrity.
   b. an expiration date.
   c. seams and filters to be sure they are intact.
   d. all the above.

4. Hydrogen peroxide is an effective sterilizing agent for linens and gauze sponges.
   a. True
   b. False

5. Implantable devices
   a. should be immediate use steam sterilized in extended cycles.
   b. should only be sterilized using ethylene oxide.
   c. should not be immediate use steam sterilized unless there is a tracking system in place to trace the item to a patient.
   d. should be discarded if not used.

6. One common cause of a clogged drain screen is
   a. tape.
   b. wrapper particles.
   c. poor steam quality.
   d. a malfunctioning baffle plate.

7. The best way to clean a suction lumen is
   a. using running warm water.
   b. using the proper sized brush.
   c. soaking in an enzyme solution for three minutes.
   d. using the appropriate stylet.

197

8. Which of the following statements about endoscopes is true?
   a. Not all endoscopes can be processed in an automated endoscope reprocessor.
   b. Ultrasonic cleaning is the process of choice for endoscopes.
   c. Flexible endoscopes are not easily damaged.
   d. All endoscopes should be steam sterilized.

9. When using high-level disinfectants it is important to remember that they may be deactivated by
   a. dilution.
   b. organic matter.
   c. time.
   d. all the above.

10. Which of the following steps happens first when processing flexible endoscopes?
    a. Leak testing
    b. High-level disinfecting/sterilizing
    c. Manual cleaning
    d. Drying

11. All rigid sterilization containers have tamper-evident seals.
    a. True
    b. False

12. Tissue forceps have teeth.
    a. True
    b. False

13. Under current regulations who is required to report suspected medical device-related deaths to the U.S. Food and Drug Administration?
    a. Device manufacturer
    b. Hospitals
    c. All of the above
    d. None of the above

14. Floors in the Central Service department should be
    a. wet-mopped daily.
    b. wet-mopped weekly.
    c. swept daily and wet-mopped weekly.
    d. swept daily. Sweeping stirs dust

15. The staining method most frequently used to identify the shape and characteristics of bacteria is called
    a. acid fast.
    b. Ziehl Neelsen.
    c. gram.
    d. skin test.

3

198

16. During instrument manufacture the process of passivation helps build a protective chromium oxide layer on the instrument's surface.
    a. True
    b. False

17. The first step to inspect the insulation of a laparoscopic instrument is to
    a. check the collar at the distal tip.
    b. try to slide the insulation back.
    c. check the handle for chipping or cracking.
    d. visually check the instrument's shaft.

18. When arranging paper/plastic pouches in the sterilizer, the pouches should be arranged
    a. paper-to-plastic.
    b. paper-to-paper.
    c. plastic-to-plastic.
    d. the way in which the most packages can be placed in the sterilizer.

19. Items that are introduced directly into the bloodstream or other normally sterile areas of the body are classified as
    a. critical items.
    b. semi-critical items.
    c. non-critical items.
    d. equipment.

20. The first sink bay in the decontamination area should be filled with a neutral detergent or enzyme.
    a. True
    b. False

21. Regulations under the Clean Air Act are administered by the
    a. Occupational Safety and Health Administration.
    b. U.S. Food and Drug Administration.
    c. Environmental Protection Agency.
    d. Association of periOperative Registered Nurses.

22. If soiled items are held in user units before pick up for processing, they must be kept at the patient's bedside until Central Service collects them.
    a. True
    b. False

23. Jewelry should not be worn in the Central Service department work areas because
    a. they harbor bacteria.
    b. they are expensive.
    c. they may be damaged.
    d. they may be misplaced or stolen.

24. One goal of point-of-use preparation is to prevent instruments from being damaged.
    a. True
    b. False

25. During handwashing, hands should be lathered and scrubbed for at least
    a. 10 seconds.
    b. 20 seconds.
    c. one minute.
    d. two minutes.

26. All bacteria require the same conditions to live and grow.
    a. True
    b. False

27. The term *oscopy* means
    a. visual examination.
    b. disease.
    c. surgical removal.
    d. diagnosis of a medical condition.

28. Instrument sets and other required instrumentation needed for all scheduled procedures for an entire day are usually pulled
    a. two days before they will be used.
    b. the day or evening before they will be used.
    c. the morning of the planned surgery.
    d. early morning (for morning procedures) and early afternoon (for afternoon procedures) on the day of surgery.

29. A *septoplasty* is
    a. the repair of the small intestine.
    b. repair of a septic wound.
    c. repair of a tendon sheath.
    d. straightening the nose.

30. Personal protective equipment is not required when cleaning items for immediate use steam sterilization.
    a. True
    b. False

31. The weakest part of a steam sterilizer is the
    a. jacket.
    b. gasket.
    c. door.
    d. thermostatic valve.

32. Because shelf life is event related, stock rotation is no longer necessary.
    a. True
    b. False

33. Aluminum foil is an approved packaging material for use in ethylene oxide sterilizers.
    a. True
    b. False

cannot be fixed

can be replaced or repaired

34. Stainless steel jaw needle holders last longer than tungsten carbide jaw needle holders.
    a. True
    b. False

35. Endoscopes are often processed in a mechanical unit called
    a. an ultrasonic cleaner.
    b. a washer-disinfector.
    c. a flush-pulse endoscope reprocessor.
    d. an automatic endoscope reprocessor.

36. Which of the following is NOT an acceptable sterilization packaging material?
    a. Muslin
    b. Barrier cloth
    c. Canvas
    d. Twills

37. Phenolics are classified as
    a. intermediate- to low-level disinfectants.
    b. intermediate- to high-level disinfectants.
    c. high-level disinfectants.
    d. sterilants.

38. Cleaning is defined as the removal of all visible and non-visible soil.
    a. True
    b. False

39. Standards and regulations help set
    a. minimal levels of quality and safety.
    b. equal pay practices.
    c. productivity time lines.
    d. all of the above.

40. When it is necessary to transport soiled items between facilities using a truck or van, facilities must consult U.S. Department of Transportation, as well as state and local laws for transporting biohazardous items.
    a. True
    b. False

41. Which of the following is NOT a requirement of the Occupational Safety and Health Administration Bloodborne Pathogen Standard?
    a. Provide hepatitis B vaccine to employees at no cost
    b. Observe standard precautions
    c. Keep biohazard areas locked
    d. Use engineering controls to prevent biohazard exposures

42. Due to the difficulty of cleaning items contaminated with prions
    a. disposable instrument should be used during the case.
    b. heat sensitive items should not be used as they will probably be destroyed during cleaning.
    c. if reusable items are used guidelines suggest disposing of the items contaminated with high risk tissue.
    d. all the above.

43. Arthroscopy means
    a. visual exam of a joint.
    b. surgical replacement of a joint.
    c. inflammation of a joint.
    d. surgical removal of a joint.

44. The hip joint is an example of a
    a. gliding joint.
    b. ball and socket joint.
    c. pivot joint.
    d. hinge joint.

45. All items sterilized or high-level disinfected at the point of use must be carefully monitored and logged.
    a. True
    b. False

46. When loading a steam sterilizer
    a. basin sets should be placed on edge and tilted.
    b. solid containers should be placed so air can get out.
    c. there should be visible space between packs.
    d. do all of the above.

47. One of the goals of stock arrangement is to provide minimal product handling while allowing first in, first out rotation.
    a. True
    b. False

48. What exposure monitoring is required for all personnel using a hydrogen peroxide sterilizer?
    a. No monitoring is required
    b. Daily
    c. Semi annually
    d. Monthly

49. To properly test the sharpness of scissors four inches or less use
    a. yellow test material.
    b. red test material.
    c. an index cart.
    d. orange test material.

50. Loaner instrumentation can cause receiving challenges.
    a. True
    b. False

51. When placing instruments in a peel pack, the tips should always face the paper side of the pack.
    a. True
    b. False

52. When mixing several low- to intermediate-level disinfectants together, it is important to remember
    a. they should be mixed in a well-ventilated room.
    b. the mixture must be tested for its minimum effective concentration before use.
    c. nitrile gloves should be used to protect your hands.
    d. chemicals should not be mixed.

53. Powered surgical instruments should be cleaned using a mechanical cleaning process.
    a. True
    b. False

54. Following Occupational Safety and Health Administration regulations for wearing personal protective equipment in the Central Service decontamination area is optional.
    a. True
    b. False

55. It is acceptable to transport soiled and clean items at the same time in the same cart if they are placed on separate shelves.
    a. True
    b. False

56. What color should biohazard labels/signs be?
    a. Red/orange
    b. Orange/yellow
    c. Orange/blue
    d. Green/black

57. Microorganisms reproduce by a process called
    a. repopulation.
    b. binary fission.
    c. replication.
    d. bilateral reproduction.

58. Not understanding medical terminology may compromise patient care.
    a. True
    b. False

59. This the first step in the sterilization process.
    a. Receiving
    b. Sorting
    c. Soaking
    d. Cleaning

60. This surgical procedure is the removal of the gall bladder.
    a. Cholecystectomy
    b. Colectomy
    c. Parotidectomy
    d. Gastrectomy

61. When transporting items that have been immediate use steam sterilized, it is required that
    a. they be transported in a closed container.
    b. they be transported to the patient area within five minutes of the completion of the sterilization cycle.
    c. they be allow to properly cooled before transport.
    d. they be transported in such a manner that reduces the potential for contamination.

62. Using the wrong container filter or poor filter placement can be a cause of a wet pack.
    a. True
    b. False

63. Heavy items should be placed
    a. on the shelf first.
    b. on the bottom shelf.
    c. on the middle shelves.
    d. on the lower shelves.

64. Lumens should be moist when using hydrogen peroxide as a sterilizing agent.
    a. True
    b. False

65. Outside shipping containers
    a. should be removed prior to placing the items in storage.
    b. may be stored in the sterile storage area as long as they are not stored near the in house sterilized items.
    c. make good storage containers to help keep items from falling from the shelves.
    d. all the above.

66. Microgrind or supercut scissors are usually identified with a black handle.
    a. True
    b. False

67. The purpose of the insulation covering laparoscopy instruments is to
    a. protect the surgeon from burns.
    b. it helps keep the instrument from slipping during surgery.
    c. protect the patient from electrical current.
    d. protect the patient from cauterization.

68. Airflow in the prep and pack area should be
    a. negative.
    b. positive.
    c. at least four exchanges per hour.
    a. from the decontamination area to the preparation and packaging area.

69. The process by which all forms of microorganisms are completely destroyed is called
    a. high-level disinfection.
    b. thermal disinfection.
    c. sterilization.
    d. chemical disinfection.

70. What is the most common pH for detergents used for most cleaning processes?
    a. low pH.
    b. high pH.
    c. neutral pH.
    d. It depends on the water temperature and exposure time.

71. Surgical instruments are carefully inspected for cleanliness and function in the _____ area of the Central Service department.
    a. decontamination
    b. sterilization   *All Items are in sterile wrap*
    c. sterile storage
    d. preparation and packaging

72. This surgical procedure consists of removing an ear bone that has thickened and no longer transmits sound waves and replacing it with an artificial implant to improve hearing.
    a. Tympanoplasty
    b. Stapedectomy
    c. Auditory implantation
    d. Myringotomy

73. Multiple drug resistant organisms are a declining threat to patients in healthcare facilities.
    a. True
    b. False   *MRSA/-VRE*

74. The root element *gastro* refers to the
    a. colon.
    b. heart.
    c. muscles.
    d. stomach.

75. Point-of-use preparation
    a. replaces the cleaning process.
    b. begins the cleaning process.
    c. increases Operating Room turn over time.
    d. reduces Operating Room turn over time.

76. The only way to interrupt the transmission of a causative agent is to
    a. sterilize the item.
    b. wear appropriate personal protective equipment.
    c. eliminate it.
    d. involve the Occupational Safety and Health Administration.

77. Which of the following statements about Immediate Use Steam Sterilization is true?
    a. It is the sterilization method of choice for metal instruments
    b. It is recommended to be used as a primary sterilization process by the Association for the Advancement of Medical Instrumentation and the Association of periOperative Registered Nurses.
    c. It reduces turnaround time because cleaning is not required.
    d. It should be used only when there is not time to process items using the wrapped method.

78. The guidelines for sterile storages are the same for both items sterilized in house and for items purchased sterile.
    a. True
    b. False

79. Information about a device's compatibility with a specific sterilization process should be obtained from the device's manufacturer.
    a. True
    b. False

80. The higher the bioburden on an object
    a. the more difficult it will be to sterilize.
    b. the less time it will take to sterilize.
    c. the more biological tests you will need in the load.
    d. the longer it will take to cool after sterilization.

81. Sterile storage areas should
    a. have positive airflow and at least 10 air exchanges per hour.
    b. have positive airflow and at least four air exchanges per hour.
    c. have negative airflow and at least 10 air exchanges per hour.
    d. have negative airflow and at least four air exchanges per hour.

82. The part of a hemostat that locks and holds it in position is called the box lock.
    a. True
    b. False

-3

83. The purpose of a decontamination battery is to protect powered surgical instruments from fluid invasion.
    a. True
    b. False

84. Temperature in the preparation and packaging area should be
    a. below 75 degrees Fahrenheit.
    b. between 60 and 65 degrees Fahrenheit.
    c. between 68 and 73 degrees Fahrenheit.
    d. between 70 and 75 degrees Fahrenheit.

85. In an automated washer the key source of disinfection is
    a. hydrogen peroxide.
    b. water temperature.
    c. heat.
    d. disinfecting detergent.

86. Written cleaning instructions for surgical instruments should be provided by
    a. the mechanical washer manufacturer.
    b. the device manufacturer.
    c. the detergent manufacturer.
    d. the healthcare facility.

87. In the future, which of the following will more frequently become a requirement for working in a Central Service department?
    a. On-the-job training
    b. Experience
    c. Formal education
    d. Reference from facility administrator

88. More than 55% of blood is made up of this yellowish liquid.
    a. Platelets
    b. Red blood cells
    c. White blood cells
    d. Plasma

89. Bacteria that require free oxygen are called
    a. pathogenic.
    b. anaerobic.
    c. aerobic.
    d. vibrio.

90. The suffix -*ectomy* means
    a. surgical removal.
    b. inflammation.
    c. surgical revision.
    d. visual examination of organs.

91. To prevent coagulation of proteins, instruments should be pre-rinsed using
    a. cool water.
    b. warm water.
    c. a neutral detergent.
    d. a disinfectant rinse.

92. Regulations and standards provide information to help ensure
    a. quality and safety.
    b. standard guidelines for legal protection.
    c. goals for patient safety.
    d. all the above.

93. When assembling instrument trays
    a. heavier instruments should be placed on the bottom of the tray.
    b. peel packs should be place on edge on the side of the instrument pan.
    c. instrument lumens should all be dry.
    d. wicking material should be used in all trays.

94. Devices categorized as semi-critical items, must be at least _____ prior to use.
    a. high-level disinfected
    b. intermediate-level disinfected
    c. low-level disinfected
    d. sterilized

95. The human resources tool that identifies major tasks performed by persons in specific positions is called a
    a. job duty list.
    b. job specification.
    c. task summary review.
    d. job description.

96. This gland stimulates body growth.
    a. Adrenal gland
    b. Thyroid gland
    c. Pancreas
    d. Pituitary gland

97. The steam sterilization process can be affected by the design of the medical device being sterilized.
    a. True
    b. False

98. Ethylene oxide, hydrogen peroxide and ozone sterilization process must all be monitored using chemical, physical and biological monitors.
    a. True
    b. False

99. Kerrison/laminectomy rongeurs should be tested using
    a. tissue paper.
    b. a plastic dowel rod.
    c. rubber testing material.
    d. an index card.

100. Flexible endoscopes that fail a leak test may continue to be used until the break/hole impacts the scope's function.
    a. True
    b. False

PROGRESS TEST FIVE

Complete the following 140 multiple choice and true/false questions.

1. Temperature and humidity levels need to be monitored and recorded
   a. weekly, preferably daily.
   b. each shift.
   c. at least daily.
   d. at least monthly.

2. Survey readiness is the responsibility of
   a. every Central Service technician.
   b. the Central Service management team.
   c. Central Service and other various departments.
   d. the Infection Prevention and Control department.

3. Product expiration dates are located on this part of each package.
   a. Top part of the package chevron
   b. Bottom left hand side of the package
   c. Back of the package
   d. There is no standard place to look for an expiration date

4. If an equipment malfunction causes harm to patients, it should be
   a. discarded immediately.
   b. sent to the manufacturer for repairs.
   c. sequestered for inspection by Occupational Safety and Health Administration personnel.
   d. returned immediately to the Biomedical department.

5. One type of formal monitoring is watching the department's temperature and humidity levels.
   a. True
   b. False

6. Occupational Safety and Health Administration is responsible for
   a. ethylene oxide guidelines, worker safety, and the bloodborne pathogen standard.
   b. biohazard material transport safety, personal protective equipment and product labeling.
   c. prion guidelines, Safe Medical Device Act and MedWatch.
   d. sterilization safety guidelines, decontamination safety guidelines and personal protective equipment.

7. The ears are made up of three parts
   a. inner, exterior and middle.
   b. exterior, eardrum and middle.
   c. funnel, stapes and malleus.
   d. stapes, exterior and sclera.

8. The most common reason steam sterilization failure is
   a. lack of steam contact with the instrument.
   b. temperature in the sterilizer chamber.
   c. time of the conditioning phase.
   d. dry steam.

9. When using glutaraldehyde technicians should always wear latex gloves for protection.
   a. True
   b. False

10. Using latex tubing to protect delicate instrumentation is the process of choice for items to be steam sterilized.
    a. True
    b. False

11. The purpose of using a decontamination battery or hose when cleaning powered surgical instruments is
    a. to keep fluid from entering the unit.
    b. to keep functioning batteries and cords clean.
    c. to prevent electrical shock.
    d. to test the unit while cleaning.

12. Healthcare-associated infections are
    a. most likely to occur during a surgical procedure.
    b. caused by drug resistant organisms.
    c. infections without known cures.
    d. infections which occur in the course of being treated in a healthcare facility.

13. Items that have been used in patient care should be considered contaminated.
    a. True
    b. False

14. The term *excise* means
    a. to repair.
    b. to open.
    c. to cut out.
    d. examine.

15. Water must be degassed each time the ultrasonic cleaner's tank is changed because
    a. excess bubbles from filling reduce the energy of the cavitation process.
    b. excess bubbles reduce the effectiveness of the detergent.
    c. excess bubbles decrease the temperature of the tank.
    d. excess bubbles make it difficult to see items being cleaned.

16. Wrapped trays should not be stacked because
    a. it is ok to stack light weight trays but not heavy trays as the bottom.
    b. the trays will be damaged.
    c. it can cause holes in the wrapper of the bottom tray.
    d. it will cause the shelving to bend.

17. Woven reusable fabrics are the packaging products of choice for ozone sterilization.
    a. True
    b. False

18. Instrument lubrication should be performed
    a. in the decontamination area each time the instrument is cleaned.
    b. following the manufacturer's Instructions for Use.
    c. each time the instrument is dissembled.
    d. none of the above

19. Documentation is not required for items that are immediate use steam sterilized.
    a. True
    b. False

20. Microbes
    a. can be useful in food products
    b. are useful to break down sewage
    c. can produce toxins
    d. are all of the above

21. Each year, approximately _____ patients develop a healthcare-associated infection.
    a. One million
    b. Two million
    c. 700,000
    d. 500,000

22. Monitoring records must be
    a. accurate.
    b. legible.
    c. complete.
    d. all the above.

23. Always wearing personal protective equipment in the decontamination area is a quality process.
    a. True
    b. False

24. Case cart systems
    a. reduce the amount of inventory needed in user departments.
    b. are usually used in small facilities.
    c. require a duplicate cart of supplies in inventory.
    d. are an automated supply requisition system.

25. Which of the following requires preventive maintenance standards be established for medical equipment?
    a. Occupational Safety and Health Administration
    b. The Joint Commission
    c. Association for the Advancement of Medical Instrumentation
    d. Association of periOperative Registered Nurses

26. In order to reprocess single-use devices, a hospital must be able to prove the device will act the same as it did when it was first manufactured.
    a. True
    b. False

27. The iris is
    a. one of the bones in the middle ear.
    b. the colored portion of the eye.
    c. the white portion of the eye.
    d. the circular opening that controls the amount of light entering the eye.

28. Three of the main phases of a terminal steam sterilizer cycle are
    a. gravity, exposure and exhaust.
    b. pre-vacuum, exposure and exhaust.
    c. exposure, exhaust and dry.
    d. conditioning, exposure and exhaust.

29. The use of heat to kill all microorganisms, except spores, is called
    a. sterilization.
    b. thermal disinfection.
    c. high-level disinfection.
    d. mechanical disinfection.

30. Clean multi-part instruments that have been assembled to test for functionality should
    a. remain assembled for sterilization.
    b. be disassembled and placed in peel packs for sterilization.
    c. be disassembled and sterilized following manufacturer's Instructions for Use.
    d. broken down and placed in separate containers for sterilization.

31. The endoscope that would be dispensed for a procedure that required visualization of the lower part of the large intestine would be a
    a. colonoscope.
    b. sigmoidoscope.
    c. gastroscope.
    d. ureteroscope.

32. Central Service technicians must wear special attire referred to as _____ to minimize their exposure to bloodborne pathogens and other contaminants.
    a. PPE
    b. OSHA
    c. TPA
    d. CDC

33. To help prevent the growth of biofilm, soil on used instruments should be allowed to dry.
    a. True
    b. False

34. The suffix *plasty*
    a. is a prefix meaning to suture.
    b. is a prefix meaning surgical restoration.
    c. is a suffix meaning surgical restoration.
    d. means to suture.

35. Using untreated water
    a. increases the likelihood of mineral scale deposits.
    b. decreases the likelihood of mineral scale deposits.
    c. is recommended to be used during the detergent cycle.
    d. is used for the final rinse process.

36. Sterile trays should
    a. not be touched until they are properly cooled.
    b. lifted not dragged off the sterilizer cart.
    c. checked to be sure the external chemical indicators have turned the appropriate color.
    d. all the above.

37. Ethylene oxide is a toxic gas.
    a. True
    b. False

38. Scissors with tungsten carbide cutting edges are usually identified by
    a. black handles.
    b. silver handles.
    c. gold handles.
    d. the letters "TC".

39. The sterilization method of choice for single-use items is immediate use steam sterilization.
    a. True
    b. False

40. The basic unit of a living organism
    a. cells.
    b. cytoplasm.
    c. nucleus.
    d. organs.

41. Know what is dirty, know what is clean, know what is sterile; keeping the three conditions separate, and remedying contamination immediately are
    a. the principles of asepsis.
    b. the basics of the bloodborne pathogen standard.
    c. the principles of infection prevention and control.
    d. the basics of environmental control.

42. Documentation of immediate use steam sterilization cycles should include
    a. patient identification and reason for the immediate use steam sterilization cycle.
    b. leak testing results.
    c. process challenge device lot number.
    d. all the above.

43. A true Central Service quality program utilizes
    a. all Central Service personnel and a cross section of its customers.
    b. top administrators and the Infection Prevention department.
    c. surgeons and visitors.
    d. all the above.

44. Requisition systems are primarily used in large facilities.
    a. True
    b. False

45. When Central Service supports affiliated clinics
    a. only disposable instrument should be sent to the clinics.
    b. a separate tracking system must be developed for the clinic areas.
    c. planning and communication are is critical.
    d. equipment preventive maintenance and repair are not as critical.

46. Class III medical devices are identified as high risk.
    a. True
    b. False

47. An organ that filters the blood to remove amino acids and some harmful toxins
    a. kidney.
    b. pancreas.
    c. liver.
    d. gall bladder.

48. Immediate use steam sterilization is the process to sterilize trays for future use.
    a. True
    b. False

49. Which of the following are classified as high-level disinfectants?
    a. Glutaraldehyde and phenolics
    b. Glutaraldehyde and ortho-phthalaldehydes
    c. Quaternary ammonium compounds and phenolics
    d. Halogens and ortho-phthalaldehydes

50. The U.S. Food and Drug Administration classifies sterilization packaging as a
    a. Class I medical device.
    b. Class II medical device.
    c. Class III medical device.
    d. Class IV medical device.

51. Loaner instruments should
    a. be decontaminated if they appear soiled upon arrival.
    b. be sterilized using a low temperature process.
    c. be decontaminated before use.
    d. should not be used.

52. Maintaining professional conduct standards and adapting to changing situations are examples of
    a. communication abilities.
    b. teamwork.
    c. legal responsibilities.
    d. employability skills.

53. Users are responsible to notify Central Service if they discover instruments or equipment that are in need of repair.
    a. True
    b. False

54. The term *ostomy*
    a. is a prefix.
    b. is a suffix.
    c. is a root.
    d. means surgical removal.

55. Instrument lubrication is performed
    a. immediately before use.
    b. after sterilization.
    c. after cleaning.
    d. before cleaning.

56. The bottom shelf of any sterile storage system should be
    a. solid and eight to 10 inches from the floor.
    b. solid and two to four inches from the floor.
    c. cleaned weekly.
    d. wire and eight to 10 inches from the floor.

57. Cellulose-containing packaging materials are not compatible with hydrogen peroxide sterilization.
    a. True
    b. False

58. The purpose of a suction stylet is to
    a. unclog the suction during surgery.
    b. clean the suction in the decontamination area.
    c. facilitate the sterilization process.
    d. provide a measuring guide for the surgeon.

59. It is recommended to use immediate use steam sterilization to sterilize instruments contaminated with Creutzfeldt-Jakob disease after the procedure has been completed.
    a. True
    b. False

60. Bacteria that cause disease are called
    a. gram positive.
    b. gram negative.
    c. pathogens.
    d. potentially infectious.

61. Asepsis is defined as
    a. the absence of all microorganisms.
    b. the ability to prevent a healthcare-associated infection.
    c. the ability to stop the chain of infection.
    d. the absence of microorganisms that cause disease.

62. External indicators can prove an item is sterile when the sterilization cycle is complete.
    a. True
    b. False

63. The degree or grade of excellence of a product or service is called
    a. Six Sigma.
    b. Lean.
    c. the international standard organization 9000.
    d. quality.

64. Capital equipment items are items
    a. with a high cost.
    b. with a low purchase cost.
    c. that are purchased, stored, consumed and reordered.
    d. used for patient care.

65. Which of the following statements is correct?
    a. Patient care equipment tracking requires a computer
    b. Patient care equipment should only be tracked if it has a value in excess of an amount specified by the facility
    c. Tracking patient care equipment can prevent equipment shortages
    d. Patient care equipment must only be tracked if its usage will be charged to patients

66. Medical device reporting is regulated by the
    a. National Fire Protection Association.
    b. Environmental Protection Agency.
    c. World Health Organization.
    d. U.S. Food and Drug Administration.

67. This surgical procedure removes tissue or displaced bone from the wrist area to release pressure on the median nerve.
    a. Carpal tunnel repair
    b. Ulnar nerve transposition
    c. Arthrotomy
    d. Fasciotomy

68. Steam flush pressure pulse sterilizers are a type of gravity sterilizers.
    a. True
    b. False

69. Thermal disinfection is accomplished using
    a. heated chemicals.
    b. heated glutaraldehyde.
    c. prolonged high pressure steam.
    d. heat.

70. When placing instruments in a peel pack, the tips should always face the paper side of the pack.
    a. True
    b. False

71. Information regarding cleaning processes for endoscopes should be provided by
    a. the Society of Gastroenterology Nurses and Associates.
    b. Association for Professionals in Infection Control and Epidemiology.
    c. the instrument manufacturer.
    d. the operating room staff.

72. Which of the following is an advantage of minimally invasive surgery?
    a. Cost saving for the patient
    b. Shorter recovery times
    c. All procedures can be done in a same day surgery center
    d. Fewer instruments are used

73. When moving transport carts throughout the healthcare facility, Central Service technicians must always yield right of way to patients and visitors.
    a. True
    b. False

74. The last word element in a medical term is the
    a. combining vowel.
    b. prefix.
    c. suffix.
    d. root.

75. Instruments should be cleaned using a
    a. circular motion.
    b. to and fro motion.
    c. stiff metal brush.
    d. water spray.

76. Trays that overhang the shelving
    a. can become contaminated.
    b. is ok for rigid containers but not for flat wrapped trays.
    c. is an appropriate way to store trays as it allows for the use of proper body mechanics when lifting heavy trays.
    d. none of the above.

77. An extended aeration cycle is required for items sterilized in ozone sterilization processes.
    a. True
    b. False

78. Instrument marking tape should be wrapped approximately _____ around the instrument.
    a. 1.5 times
    b. two times
    c. 2.5 times
    d. three times

79. Items to be disinfected or sterilized at point of use must be
    a. properly cleaned per manufacturer's Instructions for Use.
    b. semi-critical devices.
    c. non-critical devices.
    d. all the above.

80. _____ is an example of a fungus.
    a. Pneumonia
    b. Tuberculosis
    c. Athlete's foot
    d. Herpes simplex

81. Hand hygiene means hands are kept germ free at work.
    a. True
    b. False

82. A biological indicator is called positive when
    a. the incubation process is complete.
    b. when there is no growth in the ampule after incubation.
    c. when there is growth in the ampule after incubation.
    d. prior to sterilization.

83. Quality planning includes studying other facilities.
    a. True
    b. False

84. The inventory system that stocks supplies by established stock levels is called
    a. a periodic automated replenishment system.
    b. case cart.
    c. an ADT system.
    d. exchange system.

85. All patient care equipment that was dispensed for use must be considered _____,
    and handled as such, regardless of its appearance.
    a. sterile
    b. clean
    c. contaminated
    d. visibly soiled

86. Agency which imposes very strict labeling requirements on manufacturers of chemicals
    used by Central Service departments.
    a. Occupational Safety and Health Administration
    b. U.S. Food and Drug Administration
    c. Environmental Protection Agency
    d. Association for the Advancement of Medical Instrumentation

87. The largest part of the human brain is the
    a. brain stem.
    b. cerebellum.
    c. cerebrum.
    d. spinal cord

88. The coolest place in a steam sterilizer is
    a. the gasket.
    b. the thermostatic valve.
    c. the jacket.
    d. the chamber.

89. How long must alcohol remain in wet contact with an item to achieve a reasonable level of disinfection?
    a. Three to 15 minutes
    b. Two to five minutes
    c. Five to 10 minutes
    d. 10 to 20 minutes

90. Temperatures in a sterile storage area should be 55 degrees to 60 degrees Fahrenheit.
    a. True
    b. False

91. All flexible endoscopes have internal channels.
    a. True
    b. False

92. While items may be dispensed to all areas of a facility, the major focus of the sterile storage personnel is
    a. the Emergency Department.
    b. Labor & Delivery.
    c. Materiel Management.
    d. the Operating Room.

93. The following symbolizes

    a. product lot number.
    b. use by date.
    c. single-use item (do not reuse).
    d. product manufacture date.

94. Everyone who may transport contaminated items must be trained in safe handling procedures.
    a. True
    b. False

95. The purpose of a combining vowel is to
    a. tell the primary meaning of a word.
    b. identify the meaning of the root word element.
    c. ease pronunciation of a word.
    d. connects the prefix and the suffix.

96. Instruments received from surgery and tagged for repair do not need to be cleaned until they come back from repair.
   a. True
   b. False

97. Customer surveys are ineffective tools in establishing Central Service quality processes.
   a. True
   b. False

98. Which of the following systems provides supplies and instruments for individual surgical procedures?
   a. Exchange cart
   b. Periodic automated replenishment system
   c. Case cart
   d. Requisition

99. The shelving system of choice for the sterile storage area is
   a. closed.
   b. semi closed.
   c. open.
   d. track.

100. Aluminum foil is an approved packaging material for use in ethylene oxide sterilizers.
   a. True
   b. False

101. After applying instrument identification tape, instruments should be autoclaved to help the tape bond to the instrument.
   a. True
   b. False

102. Both the Association of periOperative Registered Nurses and The Joint Commission recommend that
   a. the use of immediate use steam sterilization be minimized or decreased.
   b. immediate use steam sterilization be performed in only one sterilizer per facility.
   a. healthcare facilities get U.S. Food and Drug Administration approval for immediate use steam sterilization.
   c. only Central Service technicians operate immediate use steam sterilizers.

103. The part of a cell that controls cell function is the
   a. cytoplasm.
   b. nucleus.
   c. cell membrane.
   d. capsule.

104. When putting on personal protective equipment it is important to put the mask on first.
   a. True
   b. False

105. Washer disinfector screens should be cleaned at least
    a. daily.
    b. each shift.
    c. weekly, preferably daily.
    d. monthly.

106. The Hospital Consumer Assessment of Healthcare Providers and Systems
    a. is a government program designed to eliminate mistakes in healthcare.
    b. is designed to evaluate hospital stays from a patient's perception.
    c. is part of the international standard organization 9000 program.
    d. all the above.

107. This program is designed to reduce harm to the environment
    a. case cart system.
    b. STAT requisition.
    c. sustainability.
    d. automatic reorders.

108. The decision to use reusable or disposable instruments in procedure trays is determined by
    a. where the instruments will be used.
    b. the Infection Prevention department.
    c. several factors including physician preference, storage and cost.
    d. amount of items to be used and delivery schedules.

109. Cartilage is replaced by bone through a process called
    a. ossification.
    b. calcification.
    c. osmosis.
    d. cancellous formation.

110. The steam sterilization process can be affected by the types of soil present on the devices to be sterilized.
    a. True
    b. False

111. These chemicals are used on animate (living tissue) to slow the growth of microorganisms
    a. glutaraldehyde.
    b. disinfectants.
    c. halogens.
    d. antiseptics.

112. Cellulose materials cannot be processed within a hydrogen peroxide sterilizer.
    a. True
    b. False

113. Temperature and humidity levels in the sterile storage area should be checked and recorded at least weekly.
    a. True
    b. False

114. Ethylene oxide, hydrogen peroxide and ozone sterilization can all use the same packaging materials.
    a. True
    b. False

115. Preference cards are used with a requisition inventory system.
    a. True
    b. False

116. Preventive maintenance
    a. is performed when a piece of equipment injures a patient.
    b. is designed to identify potential problems before they occur.
    c. is performed when a user unit notices a problem.
    d. is done by Central Service before equipment is dispensed.

117. Increased education helps technicians provide higher quality services.
    a. True
    b. False

118. Which of the following common items of patient care equipment limits the development of deep vein thrombosis and peripheral edema in immobile patients?
    a. Respirator
    b. Intermittent suction device
    c. Sequential compression unit
    d. Defibrillator

119. Central Service technicians need to understand the anatomy of a steam sterilizer
    a. to know how to properly clean the chamber.
    b. to understand how the sterilizer operates.
    c. to understand how to test the thermostatic trap.
    d. to know how to properly maintain the jacket.

120. The spore is the control unit of a cell.
    a. True
    b. False

121. The main theory of standard precautions is
    a. that patients in high-risk categories may be infectious.
    b. that patients diagnosed with a specific disease may be infectious.
    c. that patients are generally healthy unless they show symptoms of an infectious disease.
    d. to treat all human blood and body fluids as infectious.

122. The International Standards Organization uses routine and unannounced inspections to monitor standards in healthcare facilities.
    a. True
    b. False

123. The U.S. Food and Drug Administration Class II chemical indicator run daily in dynamic air removal sterilizers is called
    a. process challenge device.
    b. external chemical indicator.
    c. biological indicator.
    d. Bowie-Dick test.

124. Equipment should be inspected for obvious hazards such as cracked or frayed electrical cords
    a. only by trained biomedical engineering technicians.
    b. only during preventive maintenance activities.
    c. only when there are complaints from user department personnel.
    d. whenever the equipment is inspected in Central Service.

125. Documentation log sheets should be maintained when using a high-level disinfectant.
    a. True
    b. False

126. Many words may contain more than one root element.
    a. True
    b. False

127. Horizontal work surfaces in the decontamination area should be cleaned and disinfected once per day.
    a. True
    b. False

128. Accessories for electric powered equipment include
    a. hoses.
    b. foot switches.
    c. pressure regulators.
    d. decontamination hoses.

129. The use of analytical skills to solve problems and make decisions is a component of which of the following knowledge and skills dimensions?
    a. Communication abilities
    b. Facility system responsibilities
    c. Employability skills
    d. Safety practices

130. One of the goals of point-of-use preparation and transport is to
    a. speed up the decontamination process.
    b. ensure all the instruments are returned to Central Service.
    c. prevent cross contamination.
    d. all the above.

131. Automated supply replenishment systems are
    a. no longer used.
    b. used only in surgery.
    c. difficult to manage.
    d. computerized.

132. Most powered surgical instruments are immiscible.
    a. True
    b. False

133. The sterile storage process starts
    a. when items are received in the decontamination area.
    b. after items are sterilized and cooled.
    c. when the sterilizer door is opened.
    d. when items go into the sterilizer.

134. The place where the two parts of an instrument meet and pivot is called the box lock.
    a. True
    b. False

135. When sterilizing items at point of use an abbreviated sterilization cycle may be used due to the urgent need for the instruments.
    a. True
    b. False

136. Technicians in the _____ department perform safety inspections and functional tests on equipment.
    a. Materiel Management
    b. Infection Prevention
    c. Biomedical Engineering
    d. facilities and maintenance

137. The inventory system that uses two identical carts to facilitate supply replenishment is called the
    a. case cart system.
    b. exchange cart system.
    c. periodic automated replenishment system.
    d. requisition system.

138. All department staff members must be fully engaged to make a quality program successful.
    a. True
    b. False

139. Chemical indicators can show a fail result because of
    a. sterilizer malfunction.
    b. using the wrong chemical indicator.
    c. using the wrong sterilization cycle.
    d. all the above.

140. Pyrogens
    a. are fever-producing substances.
    b. are microorganisms that have survived sterilization.
    c. cause Creutzfeldt-Jakob disease.
    d. are soil particles.

PROGRESS TEST SIX

Complete the following 175 multiple choice and true/false questions.

1. Information technology is often the cornerstone of initiatives to transform healthcare.
    a. True
    b. False

2. Disposable items increase combustible load in a healthcare facility.
    a. True
    b. False

3. Enabling people to use information gained to interact with others is known as
    a. human relations.
    b. communications.
    c. cross-functional teams.
    d. moral behavior.

4. At this time, tracking systems are unable to track worker productivity information.
    a. True
    b. False

5. A step in communication that occurs when a listener asks a question is called
    a. stereotyping.
    b. feedback.
    c. communication looping.
    d. halo interpretation.

6. Improving your professional development skills is an important part of
    a. the interview process.
    b. networking.
    c. the certification process.
    d. career advancement.

7. The U.S. Food and Drug Administration Class II chemical indicator run daily in dynamic air removal sterilizers is called a
    a. process challenge device.
    b. external chemical indicator.
    c. biological indicator.
    d. Bowie-Dick test.

8. Always wearing personal protective equipment in the decontamination area is a quality process.
    a. True
    b. False

9. Product expiration dates are located on this part of each package.
    a. Top part of the package chevron
    b. Bottom left hand side of the package
    c. Back of the package
    d. There is no standard place to look for an expiration date

10. When patient equipment enters a healthcare facility, it must be safety checked by a _____ before it is cleared for patient use.
    a. Biomedical technician
    b. infection control committee member
    c. Central Service technician
    d. Central Service director

11. These are used to breakdown fatty tissue on instruments
    a. protease enzymes.
    b. lipase enzymes.
    c. amylase enzymes.
    d. neutral pH cleaners.

12. Anaerobic bacteria require free oxygen to live.
    a. True
    b. False

13. The absence of microorganisms that cause disease is called
    a. infection prevention.
    b. infection control.
    c. asepsis.
    d. HIA control.

14. Immediate use steam sterilization was developed to process items when the facility does not have enough instruments to perform the surgery.
    a. True
    b. False

15. When an instrument has a shiny surface it is said to have a _____ finish.
    a. satin
    b. passivation
    c. matte
    d. mirror

16. Lumens should be moist when sterilized using hydrogen peroxide as a sterilizing agent.
    a. True
    b. False

17. Most Central Service departments employ some sort of automated Information management system.
    a. True
    b. False

18. Ethylene oxide gas canisters should be stored
    a. in a containment locker.
    b. outside.
    c. in a refrigerator.
    d. in a chamber heated to 75 degrees Fahrenheit.

19. Knowing what is expected and consistently meeting those expectations are part of
    a. effective communications.
    b. ethical behavior.
    c. job success.
    d. professional behavior.

20. Improving employability skills requires
    a. identifying requirements for upper-level education.
    b. creating a timeline for promotion.
    c. identifying requirements for your goal.
    d. all the above.

21. Sterile packages should be stored no lower than eight to 10 inches from the floor.
    a. True
    b. False

22. Combining vowels are used to
    a. help with the pronunciation of the word.
    b. connects two similar terms.
    c. change the meaning of the root.
    d. helps designate the term as a medical anatomy term.

23. If soiled instruments are to be transported to an offsite facility for processing
    a. they should be counted prior to placing them in the transport vehicle.
    b. they should be placed in special containers made for instrument transport.
    c. they should be transported following the U.S. or state Department of Transportation guidelines.
    d. they should be transported following the Association for Professionals in Infection Control and Epidemiology safe transportation guidelines.

24. The decontamination area of the Central Service department is where instruments are carefully checked for cleanliness and function.
    a. True
    b. False

25. Arthroscopy instruments are used during
    a. robotic surgery.
    b. laparoscopic surgery.
    c. joint surgery.
    d. all the above.

26. Some plastics including formulations of spun-bonded polyolefin are intended for use in these sterilization processes
    a. steam.
    b. ozone and hydrogen peroxide.
    c. liquid.
    d. gravity.

27. The amount of time an item must remain wet with a disinfectant to achieve disinfection is called.
    a. Holding time
    b. Wet contact time
    c. Activation
    d. Sterilization time

28. The drain screen in a steam sterilizer must be cleaned
    a. weekly, preferably daily.
    b. each cycle.
    c. at least daily.
    d. during routine preventative maintenance.

29. This surgical procedure removes the uterus.
    a. Hysteroscopy
    b. Hysterectomy
    c. Dilatation & curettage
    d. Bilateral salpingo-oophorectomy

30. Recommendations regarding sterilization practices are provided by the Association for the Advancement of Medical Instrumentation.
    a. True
    b. False

31. Which of the following is NOT a result of computer integration?
    a. Eliminating redundant entry of information
    b. Promotes efficiency
    c. Automatically provides critical update to industry standards
    d. Reduced inaccurate and conflicting information

32. A plane crash is an example of an external disaster.
    a. True
    b. False

33. Effective communication skills will resolve all communication problems.
    a. True
    b. False

34. Professional development is a commitment to continuous learning.
    a. True
    b. False

35. In addition to providing financial and operational management, information technology systems are used to help ensure patient safety.
    a. True
    b. False

36. Which of the following is true about a valuing diversity effort?
    a. It "happens" because top-level officials require it
    b. It occurs because a Central Service director desires it
    c. It is a "program" in which a committee "decides what to do"
    d. None of the above statements is correct

37. Safety relates to freedom from damage, risk or injury.
    a. True
    b. False

38. Personal development is mandatory while professional development is only needed for career advancement.
    a. True
    b. False

39. Employee training should occur
    a. for new employees.
    b. at least monthly.
    c. for employees who moves to a new position.
    d. for both new employees and employees who moves to a new position.

40. If everyone develops a quality-driven focus, written policies and procedures are not necessary in the Central Service department.
    a. True
    b. False

41. The movement of supplies throughout the healthcare facility is called
    a. distribution.
    b. inventory management.
    c. case cart system.
    d. procurement.

42. All patient care equipment that was dispensed for use must be considered _____, and handled as such, regardless of its appearance.
    a. sterile
    b. clean
    c. contaminated
    d. visibly soiled

43. What is the preferred pH for detergents used for most cleaning processes?
    a. Low pH
    b. High pH
    c. Neutral pH
    d. It depends on the water temperature and exposure time

44. All microorganisms are harmful to humans.
    a. True
    b. False

45. Inanimate objects that can transmit bacteria are called
    a. transmission devices.
    b. fomites.
    c. carriers.
    d. famiseals.

46. All items sterilized or high-level disinfected at point of use must be carefully monitored and logged.
    a. True
    b. False

47. Instrument marking tape should be wrapped approximately _____ around the instrument.
    a. 1.5 times
    b. two times
    c. 2.5 times
    d. three times

48. Hydrogen peroxide kills microorganisms by a process called oxidation.
    a. True
    b. False

49. Event related shelf life means items are safe until opened for use.
    a. True
    b. False

50. The term *ectomy* means
    a. to repair.
    b. surgical removal.
    c. inflammation.
    d. to cut.

51. The proper handling of instrumentation is the responsibility of
    a. the surgeon.
    b. the scrub technician.
    c. the Central Service technician.
    d. everyone who comes in contact with the instrumentation.

52. A pick list contains information that
    a. assists the surgeon during the procedure.
    b. is used to assemble surgery instrument sets.
    c. assists the Central Service technician select the correct supplies for the sterile storage area.
    d. identifies the supplies and instruments needed for a specific doctor and procedure.

53. After use, loaner instrumentation must be decontaminated before it is shipped back to the vendor.
    a. True
    b. False

54. Cellulose materials cannot be processed within a hydrogen peroxide sterilizer.
    a. True
    b. False

55. Which of the following would be the best choice for high-level disinfection of instruments?
    a. Phenolics
    b. Chlorine
    c. Iodophors
    d. Ortho-phthalaldehydes

56. The steam sterilization process can be affected by the design of the medical device being sterilized.
    a. True
    b. False

57. Organs are two or more cells that are similar.
    a. True
    b. False

58. Which organization writes standards relating to the processing of flexible endoscopes?
    a. The Society of Gastroenterology Nurses and Associates
    b. The Association of periOperative Registered Nurses
    c. The International Standard Organization
    d. The Association for Professionals in Infection Control and Epidemiology

59. Which of these traffic control/dress code requirements applies to the clean assembly area of Central Service?
    a. Biohazard
    b. Unrestricted
    c. Semi restricted
    d. Restricted

60. Computerized tracking systems are fast, but manual tracking systems are more effective for tracking.
    a. True
    b. False

61. Which of the following information is NOT included on a safety data sheet?
    a. Special precautions
    b. Physical data
    c. Required inventory levels
    d. Product identification

62. Customer complaints are best handled through which of the following approaches?
    a. Honesty
    b. A calm attitude
    c. Being cheerful and courteous
    d. All the above

63. Networking inside your profession can help you increase your knowledge toward advancement while networking outside your profession does not.
    a. True
    b. False

64. Which of the following is NOT a feature of an instrument tracking system?
    a. Productivity information
    b. Financial data
    c. Quality assurance information
    d. Product updates and recall information

65. This process allows a person to understand someone else's needs.
    a. Communication
    b. Human relations
    c. Feedback
    d. Moral behavior

66. Safety data sheets are provided by
    a. the Occupational Safety and Health Administration.
    b. the U.S. Food and Drug Administration.
    c. the Risk Management department.
    d. the product manufacturer.

67. One important step in preparing for an interview is
    a. reviewing the certification exam questions.
    b. developing a written response to application questions.
    c. anticipating possible interview questions.
    d. all the above.

68. Sterilizer load records should contain
    a. items and quantity sterilized.
    b. types of physical monitors utilized.
    c. preventive maintenance dates.
    d. all the above.

69. The quality method failure mode and effects analysis is a
    a. method to investigate issues after they occur to prevent future occurrences.
    b. a system recommended by surveying agencies to ensure quality.
    c. a system used in all Central Service instrument process to guarantee quality.
    d. a quality method to prevent problems before they occur.

70. A disadvantage of an exchange cart system is
    a. they do not work in emergency departments.
    b. they are used for a specific procedure only.
    c. replenishment supplies need to be ordered frequently.
    d. they require duplicate inventory.

71. Patient care equipment should be stored in a _____ condition.
    a. "ready to dispense"
    b. "ready to clean"
    c. "ready to inspect"
    d. "ready to sterilize"

72. Cleaning brushes
    a. should be cleaned and sterilized at least daily.
    b. should have metal bristles.
    c. should be one larger than the lumen to be cleaned.
    d. all the above.

73. Microbiology is the study of
    a. life.
    b. microorganisms.
    c. human immune systems.
    d. all the above.

74. The basics of aseptic technique
    a. is knowing the chain of infection.
    b. are activities that prevent infection.
    c. follow the Bloodborne Pathogen Standard.
    d. are all the above.

75. To sterilize items using immediate use steam sterilization, the item's manufacturer instructions must state the item can be sterilized using an immediate use steam sterilization cycle.
    a. True
    b. False

76. Laser finished instruments are coated with a durable protective finish that cannot be chipped or scratched.
    a. True
    b. False

77. Information about a device's compatibility with a specific sterilization process should be obtained from the device's manufacturer.
    a. True
    b. False

78. Temperatures in the sterile storage area should be 64 to 78° Fahrenheit.
    a. True
    b. False

79. The suffix -*tome* means
    a. surgical restoration.
    b. surgical fixation.
    c. to suture.
    d. cutting instrument.

80. It is acceptable to transport soiled and clean items at the same time in the same cart if they are placed on separate shelves.
    a. True
    b. False

81. Soiled instruments and other items are received in the _____ area of the Central Service department.
    a. preparation
    b. packaging
    c. decontamination
    d. sterilization

82. Which of the following should be used to thoroughly rinse (remove) all traces of disinfectant from an endoscope's channels?
    a. Forced air
    b. Water containing approved sterilant
    c. Treated water
    d. A heated glutaraldehyde

83. When placing instruments that open in an instrument tray, you should
    a. lock the handles to prevent damage during sterilization.
    b. arrange the instruments in alphabetical order.
    c. arrange the instruments in the order of their use.
    d. unlock the handles and open the instruments.

84. Items that are introduced directly into the bloodstream or other normally sterile areas of the body are classified as
    a. critical items.
    b. semi-critical items.
    c. non-critical items.
    d. equipment.

85. Gravity steam sterilizers use a pump or water injector to remove air from the chamber.
    a. True
    b. False

86. The procedure to remove the stomach is
    a. sastritis.
    b. gastrectomy.
    c. gastric bypass.
    d. gastric sleeve.

87. Failure to receive accreditation from The Joint Commission can result in the loss of Medicare and Medicaid payments.
    a. True
    b. False

88. Which of the following tracking methods provides real-time information?
    a. Radio frequency identification tags
    b. Laser-etched bar codes
    c. Standard bar codes
    d. Dot matrix applications

89. Healthcare facilities using ethylene oxide should have a dedicated ventilation system to remove residual ethylene oxide during the exhaust cycle.
    a. True
    b. False

90. Which of the following is an example of communication?
    a. The words you speak
    b. The words you write
    c. Non-verbal expressions you use
    d. All of the above

91. Professional development skill building activities include
    a. team building activities.
    b. public speaking.
    c. writing.
    d. all the above.

92. A group of employees from different departments within the healthcare facility that work together to solve operating problems is called a
    a. decision-making team.
    b. multi-dimensional team.
    c. cross-functional team.
    d. management-sub management team.

93. Which of the following is NOT a component of risk management?
    a. Injury management
    b. Claims management
    c. Staff management
    d. Accident reporting

94. Planning and reviewing your goals will help identify activities to help you meet those goals.
    a. True
    b. False

95. Documentation of immediate use steam sterilization cycles should include
    a. patient identification and reason for the immediate use steam sterilization cycle.
    b. leak testing results.
    c. process challenge device lot number.
    d. all the above.

96. Quality requires the efforts and participation of everyone in the healthcare facility.
    a. True
    b. False

97. Supplies such as disposable wraps are called
    a. consumable.
    b. capital supplies.
    c. patient care supplies.
    d. assets.

98. Preventive maintenance
    a. is performed when a piece of equipment injures a patient.
    b. is designed to identify potential problems before they occur.
    c. is performed when a user unit notices a problem.
    d. is done by Central Service before equipment is dispensed.

99. Detergents used in mechanical cleaners should be
    a. low alkaline.
    b. low acid.
    c. low temperature.
    d. low foaming.

100. When cleaning prion contaminated instruments no special cleaning procedures are required only following standard cleaning protocols and the Manufacturer's Instructions for Use.
    a. True
    b. False

101. Hand hygiene is considered the single most important factor in reducing infections.
    a. True
    b. False

102. Immediate use steam sterilization documentation should include
    a. name of the patient for which the items were sterilized.
    b. sterilizer number and cycle.
    c. name of the instrument sterilized.
    d. all the above.

103. An osteotome is
    a. used to cut or shave bone.
    b. a retractor.
    c. a hemostatic forceps.
    d. none of the above.

104. Woven reusable fabrics are the packaging products of choice for ozone sterilization.
    a. True
    b. False

105. Sterile items should be stored at least _____ inches below sprinkler heads.
    a. Eight
    b. 18
    c. 12
    d. 15

106. Which of the following means *beside* or *near*?
    a. Para
    b. Peri
    c. Parta
    d. Pana

107. Decontamination of instruments and equipment starts
    a. during the manual cleaning process.
    b. as soon as the instruments are received in the decontamination area.
    c. at the point of use.
    d. when the instruments are placed back in their trays at the point of use.

108. All Central Service departments perform the same basic services.
    a. True
    b. False

109. Leak testing should be performed on each flexible endoscope annually.
    a. True
    b. False

110. When placing instruments in a peel pack, the tips should always face the paper side of the pack.
    a. True
    b. False

111. Devices listed as critical items, must be _____ prior to use.
    a. high-level disinfected
    b. intermediate-level disinfected
    c. low-level disinfected
    d. sterilized

112. When combining loads, hard goods should be placed on the top shelves to allow for more efficient removal of the condensate.
    a. True
    b. False

113. Items that are wrapped moist can be a cause of wet packs.
    a. True
    b. False

114. A herniorrhaphy surgical procedure is
    a. repair of a shoulder muscle.
    b. repair of a muscle layer that is allowing all or part of an organ to project through an opening.
    c. removal of a sample of diseased or infected muscle.
    d. repair of fibrous membranes that cover a muscle.

115. Voluntary standards
    a. provide a guideline for required levels of service.
    b. provide guidelines for better patient care.
    c. are written enforceable guidelines.
    d. are guidelines followed by the Centers for Disease Control.

116. Tracking individual instruments is important to help ensure specific instruments are kept with a specific set.
    a. True
    b. False

117. Personal headsets should not be used in the Central Service department because they
    a. cannot be cleaned effectively.
    b. reduce the ability to hear telephones, alarms and coworkers.
    c. allow the music to be played to load potentially harming your hearing.
    d. none of the above.

118. Which of the following is NOT required for sharps safety?
    a. Dispose of all single use sharps in an appropriate container
    b. Sharp ends should be pointed away from anyone's body during transport
    c. Wash all disposable sharps before discarding them
    d. All the above are related to sharps safety

119. On the job relationships do not change when one team member has been promoted.
    a. True
    b. False

120. Hospitals can effectively validate sterilization processes.
    a. True
    b. False

121. Six Sigma focuses on
    a. reducing defects.
    b. delivering near perfect products.
    c. strives to eliminate variations in the process.
    d. all the above.

122. The following symbolizes

    a. product lot number.
    b. use by date.
    c. single-use item (do not reuse).
    d. product manufacture date.

123. The _____ requires that the healthcare facility report malfunctions of medical devices that have contributed to patient injury, illness and/or death to the manufacturer and the U.S. Food and Drug Administration.
    a. Occupational Safety and Health Administration Patient Safety Act
    b. Safe Medical Devices Act
    c. Environmental Protection Agency Patient Security Act
    d. U.S. Food and Drug Administration Equipment Notification Act

124. Because of the cavitation and impingement action of mechanical cleaners there is no need to pre-clean items that will be processed in a mechanical cleaner.
    a. True
    b. False

125. When cleaning items contaminated with pseudomonas,
    a. items should be cleaned in a separate area to prevent cross contamination.
    b. items should be placed in a disinfectant solution prior to manual cleaning.
    c. the Infection Prevention department should be notified of the contaminate.
    d. there are no special cleaning requirements for items contaminated with pseudomonas.

126. The decontamination area of the Central Service department should have
    a. a negative air flow.
    b. a positive air flow.
    c. a filtered air flow.
    d. no air exchanges because it is a biohazard area.

127. Before an item can be placed in a low-temperature sterilization processing system they must be
    a. heated.
    b. filled with air.
    c. sterilized.
    d. cleaned.

128. Stainless steel jaw needle holders last longer than tungsten carbide jaw needle holders.
    a. True
    b. False

129. Hydrogen peroxide is an effective sterilizing agent for linens and gauze sponges.
    a. True
    b. False

130. When transporting sterile items in an approved vehicle, soiled items can be transported in the same cart as long as they are on different shelves from clean or sterile items.
    a. True
    b. False

131. The term *hyster* means
    a. uterus.
    b. below.
    c. above.
    d. woman.

132. Items should be contained for transport
    a. to keep the instruments from unnecessary movement during transport.
    b. to keep the instrument sets intact.
    c. to minimize the spread of microorganisms.
    d. all the above.

133. In Central Service, the concept of "one-way flow of materials" refers to the movement of products
    a. from Central Service to surgical areas.
    b. from surgical areas to Central Service.
    c. from soiled areas to clean processing areas within Central Service.
    d. from clean processing areas to soiled areas in Central Service.

134. The muscular system
    a. assists with movement.
    b. produces heat for the body.
    c. pumps blood throughout the body.
    d. is all of the above.

135. U.S. Food and Drug Administration Medical Device recall
    a. means the items(s) cannot be used and must be pulled off the shelves.
    b. means the item(s) need to be checked or repaired.
    c. is a mandatory statute issued on a defective product.
    d. is a voluntary statute issued on a potentially defective product.

136. Endoscope cameras are sealed instruments so fluid invasion is not a concern during the cleaning process.
    a. True
    b. False

137. The U.S. Food and Drug Administration classifies sterilization packaging as a
    a. Class I Medical Device
    b. Class II Medical Device
    c. Class III Medical Device
    d. Class IV Medical Device

138. The relative humidity of the assembly area should be
    a. less than 75%.
    b. 30% to 60%.
    c. 40% to 70%.
    d. less than 35%.

139. The use of test strips to test the minimum effective concentration in high-level disinfection solutions is required
    a. weekly preferably daily.
    b. daily.
    c. each time the solution will be used.
    d. only when manual soaking systems are used.

140. After sterilization the load contents may take two hours or more to cool.
    a. True
    b. False

141. Which of the following is the most important factor necessary for teamwork?
    a. Attitude
    b. Promptness
    c. Loyalty
    d. Cooperation

142. Information about chemical or hazardous substances must be available to all employees.
    a. True
    b. False

143. The following resources will help you stay current in the Central Service field.
    a.   Conferences
    b.   On-the-job training
    c.   Continuing education
    d.   All of the above

144. A biological indicator that is incubated without being sterilized is called
    a.   positive.
    b.   negative.
    c.   a process challenge device.
    d.   control.

145. Not following established policies and procedures will result in a lower quality program.
    a.   True
    b.   False

146. Capital equipment items are
    a.   usually used for patient care.
    b.   items with a lower purchase cost.
    c.   items with a higher purchase cost.
    d.   purchased, stored, consumed and reordered.

147. Equipment leasing and rental differ in that
    a.   leasing involves purchase; rental does not require ownership.
    b.   equipment rental is usually done on a shorter-term basis than equipment leasing.
    c.   equipment leasing involves the most expensive equipment; equipment rental involves less expensive equipment.
    d.   equipment leasing is an operating expense; equipment rental does not have cost implications.

148. Powered surgical instruments
    a.   cannot be immersed.
    b.   can be immersed.
    c.   should be thoroughly cleaned at the point of use.
    d.   should be cleaned using a mechanical washer.

149. Prions are
    a.   abnormal forms of protein.
    b.   gram positive bacillus.
    c.   a type of virus.
    d.   an acid fast microorganism.

150. To protect themselves from splashes and spills, Central Service technicians assigned to the decontamination area should wear
    a.   double-cloth gowns.
    b.   blue surgical scrubs.
    c.   fluid-resistant gowns.
    d.   sterile operating room gowns.

151. When transporting items that have been immediate use steam sterilized, it is required that
    a. they be transported in a closed container.
    b. they be transported to the patient area within five minutes of the completion of the sterilization cycle.
    c. they be allow to properly cooled before transport.
    d. they be transported in such a manner that reduces the potential for contamination.

152. Instruments with tungsten carbide jaws can be easily identified by
    a. the diamond serration pattern on the instrument jaws.
    b. the black handles on the instrument.
    c. the gold handles on the instrument.
    d. the self-retaining lock on the instrument shaft.

153. Exposure monitoring is _____ for all personnel using a hydrogen peroxide sterilizer.
    a. not required
    b. required daily
    c. required semi-annually
    d. required monthly

154. All items should be removed from storage shelves prior to cleaning the shelf.
    a. True
    b. False

155. The term *ante* means
    a. against.
    b. apart.
    c. before.
    d. without.

156. Endoscopes should be cleaned and the internal channels left moist for storage.
    a. True
    b. False

157. Gauze squares are the wicking material of choice for instrument sets.
    a. True
    b. False

158. Pasteurizers disinfect using
    a. heated water.
    b. phenols.
    c. high-level disinfectants.
    d. peracetic acid.

159. When loading a steam sterilizer, basins should be
    a. placed in an upright position.
    b. loaded first.
    c. placed on edge.
    d. placed in a wire basket.

160. This tissue covers the body's external surface.
    a. Epithelial tissue
    b. Connective tissue
    c. Muscular tissue
    d. Nervous tissue

161. U.S. Food and Drug Administration recalls may be either mandatory or voluntary.
    a. True
    b. False

162. Central Service technicians who do not think they are being treated appropriately by their employer should
    a. find another job.
    b. discuss the problem with their workplace peers.
    c. discuss the situation with their supervisor.
    d. accept the situation as "the way things are done" at the facility.

163. Healthcare facilities are required by the _____ to provide adequate ventilation systems, personal protective equipment and safe work operating procedures?
    a. Environmental Protection Agency
    b. U.S. Food and Drug Administration
    c. Occupational Safety and Health Administration
    d. Centers for Medicare and Medicaid Services

164. Steps toward attaining professional goals in Central Service include
    a. certification
    b. educational conferences
    c. professional groups
    d. all the above

165. There are currently no methods available to verify cleaning process outcomes.
    a. True
    b. False

166. Viruses use this method of transportation to move.
    a. Droplet
    b. Direct contact
    c. Airborne method
    d. Viruses have no means of movement on their own

167. The best way to clean a suction lumen is
    a. using running warm water.
    b. using the proper sized brush.
    c. soaking in an enzyme solution for three minutes.
    d. using the appropriate stylet.

168. Jewelry is discouraged in sterile storage because it can damage or contaminate packages.
    a. True
    b. False

169. Automatic endoscope reprocessors are not recommended for flexible endoscopes.
   a. True
   b. False

170. When using high-level disinfectants it is important to remember they may be deactivated by
   a. dilution.
   b. organic matter.
   c. time.
   d. all the above.

171. Peel pouches should be placed _____ for sterilization.
   a. on edge, paper to plastic
   b. on edge, plastic to plastic
   c. placed flat with the plastic side up
   d. placed flat with the paper side up

172. The brain center of a cell is called the
   a. cell membrane.
   b. cytoplasm.
   c. nucleus.
   d. DNA.

173. Coaching is an example of
   a. informal communication.
   b. discipline.
   c. formal communication.
   d. mentoring.

174. The process of changing work or working conditions to reduce physical stress is
   a. called ergonomics.
   b. an employee injury reduction plan.
   c. the Occupational Safety and Health Administration Workers' Rights Program.
   d. the Occupational Safety and Health Administration's Risk Management Program.

175. When water is seen on the outside of a pack after sterilization the pack is considered safe to use if all other packs in the load are dry.
   a. True
   b. False

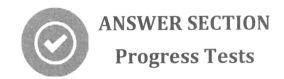

ANSWER SECTION

Progress Tests

1. A pick list contains information that
    d. *identifies the supplies and instruments needed for a specific doctor and procedure.* *(1 / 13)*

2. The basic unit of a living organism.
    a. *Cell* *(4 / 71)*

3. What is the name of the surgical procedure where an opening is made into the skull?
    b. *Craniotomy* *(3 / 45)*

4. The decontamination area of the Central Service department is where instruments are carefully checked for cleanliness and function.
    b. *False* *(1 / 10)*

5. The term "periosteal elevator" means
    d. *an instrument used to remove tissue around the bone.* *(2 / 33)*

6. Viruses
    d. *have no means of movement on their own.* *(4 / 78)*

7. The sterile storage area in a Central Service department should be restricted to
    d. *properly attired personnel meeting facility requirements.* *(1 / 14)*

8. The abbreviation *BKA* refers to a surgical procedure involving
    c. *surgical removal of the leg below the knee.* *(2 / 34)*

9. The body's control center is the
    b. *central nervous system.* *(3 / 49)*

10. The prefix word element
    b. *comes before the root.* *(2 / 23)*

11. The muscular system
    d. *is all of the above.* *(3 / 47)*

12. Microbes
    d. *are all of the above.* *(4 / 71)*

13. Prefix, suffix and roots are called word elements and are contained in all medical terms.
    b. *False* *(2 / 24)*

14. The pupil of the eye is the
    d. *circular opening that controls the amount of light entering the eye.* *(3 / 50)*

15. Skin is a type of connective tissue.
    b. *False* *(3 / 43)*

16. An advantage of centralizing Central Service management is
    c. *allows for maximization of people and services.* *(1 / 9)*

17. Prions are
    a. *abnormal forms of protein.* *(4 / 81)*

18. A herniorrhaphy is a surgical procedure which
    b. *repairs a muscle layer that is allowing all or part of an organ to project through an opening.* (3 / 48)

19. The abbreviation *CR* relates to a surgical procedure for
    a. *treating a fractured bone without a surgical incision.* (2 / 34)

20. Bacteria which cause disease are called
    c. *pathogens.* (4 / 71)

Progress Test Two   *chapter/page*

1. The U.S. Food and Drug Administration is responsible for
   d. *ensuring food, drugs and cosmetics are safe for use.* (5 / 87)

2. The basics of aseptic technique is
   b. *activities that prevent infection.* (6 / 104)

3. The decontamination area of the Central Service department should have
   a. *negative air flow.* (6 / 112)

4. Decontamination of instruments and equipment starts
   c. *at the point of use.* (7 / 121)

5. The decontamination area should have
   a. *negative air flow in relation to the other areas of the department.* (8 / 132)

6. The proper handling of instrumentation is the responsibility of
   d. *everyone who comes in contact with the instrumentation.* (7 / 122)

7. Centers for Disease Control guidelines are considered regulatory guidelines.
   b. *False* (5 / 90)

8. One of the goals of point-of-use preparation and transport is to
   c. *prevent cross contamination.* (7 / 120)

9. Automatic washers clean using a spray-force action called impingement.
   a. *True* (8 / 141)

10. The federal program designed for the voluntary reporting of device related problems is called
    d. *MedWatch.* (5 / 88)

11. When removing personal protective equipment you should remove _____ first.
    d. *shoe covers* (6 / 109)

12. Which of the following tells a primary meaning of a word?
    b. *Root word element* (2 / 23)

13. In Central Service, the concept of "one-way flow of materials" refers to the movement of products
    c. *from soiled areas to clean processing areas within Central Service.* (1 / 10)

14. Which of these traffic control/dress code requirements applies to the clean assembly area of Central Service?
    c. Semi restricted   (6 / 110)

15. End of procedure point-of-use guideline include removing gross soil, disassembling of multi-part instruments, and ensuring instruments are kept moist.
    a. True   (7 / 122-23)

16. The Association of peri-Operative Registered Nurses is
    d. a professional organization that writes guidelines for the Operating Room.   (5 / 96)

17. When putting on personal protective equipment it is important to put the mask on first.
    b. False   (6 / 109)

18. To prevent aerosols, items should be brushed below the surface of the water.
    a. True   (8 / 153)

19. The suffix -ectomy means
    b. surgical removal   (2 / 28)

20. This surgical procedure removes the uterus.
    b. Hysterectomy   (3 / 56)

21. When cleaning prion contaminated instruments no special cleaning procedures are required only following standard cleaning protocols and the Manufacturer's Instructions for Use.
    b. False   (4 / 82)

22. Healthy people do not harbor or transmit bacteria.
    b. False   (4 / 71)

23. When cleaning items contaminated with pseudomonas
    d. there are no special cleaning requirements for items contaminated
       with pseudomonas.   (4 / 78)

24. The purpose of learning medical terminology is
    c. to provide the Operating Room and medical staff with the goods and
       services they need.   (2 / 33)

25. Which organization conducts onsite survey of healthcare facilities?
    d. The Joint Commission   (5 / 97)

26. All Central Service departments perform the same basic services.
    b. False   (1 / 9)

27. Knowing and understanding medical terminology helps technicians
    c. understand what is asked when a request is made.   (2 / 22)

28. Hypoglycemia means
    c. low blood sugar.   (2 / 32)

29. If soiled instruments are to be transported to an offsite facility for processing
    c. they should be transported following the U.S. or state Department of
       Transportation guidelines.   (7 / 127)

30. All mechanical cleaning equipment provides
    c. *consistent process.* *(8 / 139)*

31. Microbiology is the study of
    b. *microorganisms.* *(4 / 70)*

32. Detergents used in mechanical cleaners should be
    d. *low foaming.* *(8 / 148)*

33. Which of the following is NOT a growing trend in Central Service?
    a. *Decentralization of Central Service responsibilities* *(1 / 9)*

34. Subcutaneous means
    c. *beneath the skin.* *(2 / 32)*

35. Spores help some microorganisms survive in adverse conditions.
    a. *True* *(4 / 73)*

36. Which of the following surgical abbreviations might be used relating to a fractured bone?
    c. *ORIF* *(2 / 35)*

37. Only good oral and written communication skills are necessary to provide or obtain information.
    b. *False* *(1 / 15)*

38. Soiled instruments and other items are received in the _____ area of the Central service department.
    c. *decontamination* *(1 / 10)*

39. A system is
    a. *a group of organs.* *(3/ 43)*

40. The procedure to remove the stomach
    b. *gastrectomy.* *(3/ 61)*

Progress Test Three *chapter/page*

1. The system used to categorize patient care items based on the degree of risk of infection.
    c. *Spaulding Classification System* *(9 / 162)*

2. An osteotome is
    a. *used to cut or shave bone.* *(10 / 182)*

3. When returning loaner items to the vendor
    c. *all items should be cleaned and decontaminated.* *(11 / 241)*

4. The first goal of creating an instrument pack is
    c. *create a pack that meets user needs.* *(12 / 246)*

5. Positive air flow means when the door is opened, air flows out of instead of into the area.
    a. *True* *(12 / 244)*

6. Molds, mushrooms and yeast are common
    b. *fungi.* *(4 / 80)*

7. The surgery of the ear that reconstructs the eardrum so sound waves can be sent to the middle ear
    a. *tympanoplasty.* *(3 / 53)*

8. Dark areas on the lens of an endoscope are?
    d. *Damaged light fibers* *(11 / 212)*

9. Soiled instruments and other items are received in the _____ area of the Central Service department.
    c. *decontamination* *(1 / 10)*

10. Pasteurizers disinfect using
    a. *heated water.* *(9 / 174)*

11. Which of the following statements about the use of mechanical washers is NOT true?
    d. *All items should be washed on the same cycle* *(8 / 144)*

12. Agency which may intervene in a matter of worker protection even if there are no specific regulations covering the situation.
    a. *Occupational Safety and Health Administration* *(5 / 93)*

13. Laser finished instruments are coated with a durable protective finish that cannot be chipped or scratched.
    b. *False* *(10 / 200)*

14. Healthcare-associated infections are
    d. *those which occur in the course of being treated in a healthcare facility.* *(1/ 18)*

15. Viruses are larger than bacteria.
    b. *False* *(4 / 78)*

16. The system that gives the body shape and support
    c. *skeletal system.* *(3 / 43)*

17. Devices categorized as semi-critical items, must be at least _____ prior to use.
    a. *high-level disinfected* *(9 / 162)*

18. Electronic testing of laparoscopic insulation should be done
    b. *in the clean assembly area prior to set assembly.* *(11 / 218)*

19. Count sheets
    c. *provide a detailed list of tray contents.* *(12 / 247)*

20. Central Service technicians must wear special attire referred to as _____ to minimize their exposure to bloodborne pathogens and other contaminants.
    a. *PPE* *(1 / 11)*

21. The temperature in the decontamination area should be between
    c. *60 to 65 degrees Fahrenheit.* *(8 / 132)*

22. Staphylococcus is classified as a gram-positive bacteria.
    a. True   *(4 / 74)*

23. Kerrison/laminectomy rongeurs should be tested using
    d. an index card.   *(10 / 196)*

24. Which of the following should be used to thoroughly rinse (remove) all traces of disinfectant from an endoscope's channels?
    c. Treated water   *(11 / 225)*

25. The prefix *hemi-*
    c. means half.   *(2 / 33)*

26. The term *septorhinoplasty* means
    b. surgical repair of the nose.   *(2 / 25)*

27. Powered surgical instrument air hoses should be pressurized for proper inspection.
    a. True   *(11 / 207)*

28. The use of test strips to test the minimum effective concentration in high-level disinfection solutions is required
    c. each time the solution will be used.   *(9 / 175)*

29. Arthroscopy instruments are used during
    c. joint surgery.   *(11 / 219)*

30. The term *itis* means
    b. inflammation.   *(2 / 27)*

31. Bacteria that do not require free oxygen to live are called
    b. anaerobic.   *(4 / 75)*

32. Instruments with tungsten carbide jaws can be easily identified by
    c. the gold handles on the instrument.   *(10 / 186)*

33. Robotic instruments
    d. are all of the above.   *(11 / 219)*

34. An important reason for instrument preparation to begin at the point of use is
    b. it helps prolong the life of the instruments.   *(7 / 121)*

35. The mechanical process by which an ultrasonic cleaner works is called cavitation.
    a. True   *(8 / 139)*

36. Clean multi-part instruments that have been assembled to test for functionality should
    c. be disassembled and sterilized following Manufacturer's Instructions for Use. *(12 / 249)*

37. To protect themselves from splashes and spills, Central Service technicians assigned to the decontamination area should wear
    c. fluid-resistant gowns.   *(6 / 108)*

38. These are used to breakdown fatty tissue on instruments
    b. lipase enzymes.   *(8 / 146)*

39. This is the lining of the uterus.
    b. *Endometrium*   *(3 / 55)*

40. Healthcare regulations and standards provide consistency of departmental activities
    by outlining
    a. *minimal levels of quality and safety.*   *(5 / 86)*

41. When a soiled instrument is found during the assembly process
    d. *the instrument and the tray it was in should be sent to the decontamination
    area for re-cleaning.*   *(12 / 249)*

42. Skeletal muscles
    b. *move only when we want them to move.*   *(3 / 47)*

43. The virus that causes hepatitis B is transmitted by
    b. *blood.*   *(4 / 78)*

44. Departmental dress codes apply to
    a. *everyone entering the Central Service department.*   *(6 / 108)*

45. All sonic cleaners have a decontamination cycle.
    b. *False*   *(8 / 139)*

46. Chemical indicators are _____ devices.
    b. *FDA Class II*   *(5 / 87)*

47. The main theory of standard precautions is
    d. *to treat all human blood and body fluids as infectious.*   *(6 / 103)*

48. Failure to perform soiled pick up rounds as scheduled can lead to instrument and
    equipment shortages.
    a. *True*   *(7 / 126)*

49. Rigid container filter retention plates should be
    a. *removed from the container and lid and cleaned separately.*   *(8 / 151)*

50. The absence of microorganisms that cause disease is called
    c. *asepsis.*   *(6 / 104)*

51. The amount of time an item must remain wet with a disinfectant to achieve
    disinfection is called
    b. *wet contact time.*   *(9 / 173)*

52. When an instrument has a shiny surface it is said to have a _____ finish.
    d. *mirror*   *(10 / 183)*

53. The word *laminectomy* means
    b. *removal of part of a lamina.*   *(2 / 28)*

54. Recommendations regarding sterilization practices are provided by the Association
    for the Advancement of Medical Instrumentation.
    a. *True*   *(5 / 95)*

55. Hand hygiene is considered the single most important factor in reducing infections.
   a. True (6 / 105)

56. Contaminated items may be returned to Central Service
   d. all the above. (7 / 121)

57. Sometimes state or local regulations differ from federal regulations and when that happens, the most stringent regulations apply.
   a. True (5 / 95)

58. Items should be contained for transport
   c. to minimize the spread of microorganisms. (7 / 124)

59. Cleaning brushes
   a. should be cleaned and sterilized at least every daily. (8 / 137)

60. The term *hypo* means
   c. below. (2 / 32)

Progress Test Four   *chapter/page*

1. The process by which instruments are sterilized for immediate use is called
   b. *Immediate Use Steam Sterilization.* (13 / 292)

2. Steam sterilization is the most commonly used method of sterilization used in healthcare because
   a. *cycles are fast and inexpensive.* (14 / 302)

3. When placing sterile items on the shelf you should check
   d. *all the above.* (16 / 350)

4. Hydrogen peroxide is an effective sterilizing agent for linens and gauze sponges.
   b. *False* (15 / 331)

5. Implantable devices
   c. *should not be immediate use steam sterilized unless there is a tracking system in place to trace the item to a patient.* (13 / 294)

6. One common cause of a clogged drain screen is
   a. *tape.* (14 / 312)

7. The best way to clean a suction lumen is
   b. *using the proper sized brush.* (10 / 154)

8. Which of the following statements about endoscopes is true?
   a. *Not all endoscopes can be processed in an automated endoscope reprocessor.* (11 / 228)

9. When using high-level disinfectants it is important to remember that they may be deactivated by
   d. *all the above.* (9 / 167)

10. Which of the following steps happens first when processing flexible endoscopes?

    a. Leak testing   *(11 / 223)*

11. All rigid sterilization containers have tamper-evident seals.

    a. True   *(12 / 284)*

12. Tissue forceps have teeth.

    a. True   *(10 / 186)*

13. Under current regulations who is required to report suspected medical device-related deaths to the U.S. Food and Drug Administration?

    c. All of the above   *(5 / 88)*

14. Floors in the Central Service department should be

    a. wet-mopped daily.   *(6 / 114)*

15. The staining method most frequently used to identify the shape and characteristics of bacteria is called

    c. gram.   *(4 / 73)*

16. During instrument manufacture the process of passivation helps build a protective chromium oxide layer on the instrument's surface.

    a. True   *(10 / 183)*

17. The first step to inspect the insulation of a laparoscopic instrument is to

    a. check the collar at the distal tip.   *(11 / 217)*

18. When arranging paper/plastic pouches in the sterilizer, the pouches should be arranged

    a. paper-to-plastic.   *(12 / 287)*

19. Items that are introduced directly into the bloodstream or other normally sterile areas of the body are classified as

    a. critical items.   *(9 / 162)*

20. The first sink bay in the decontamination area should be filled with a neutral detergent or enzyme.

    a. True   *(8 / 135)*

21. Regulations under the Clean Air Act are administered by the

    c. Environmental Protection Agency.   *(5 / 92)*

22. If soiled items are held in user units before pick up for processing, they must be kept at the patient's bedside until Central Service collects them.

    b. False   *(7 / 121)*

23. Jewelry should not be worn in the Central Service department work areas because

    a. they harbor bacteria.   *(6 / 106)*

24. One goal of point-of-use preparation is to prevent instruments from being damaged.

    a. True   *(7 / 120)*

25. During handwashing, hands should be lathered and scrubbed for at least

    b. 20 seconds.   *(6 / 105)*

26. All bacteria require the same conditions to live and grow.
    b. *False* *(4 / 75)*

27. The term *oscopy* means
    a. *visual examination.* *(2 / 28)*

28. Instrument sets and other required instrumentation needed for all scheduled procedures for an entire day are usually pulled
    b. *the day or evening before they will be used.* *(1 / 13)*

29. A *septoplasty* is
    d. *straightening the nose.* *(3 / 60)*

30. Personal protective equipment is not required when cleaning items for immediate use steam sterilization.
    b. *False* *(13 / 295)*

31. The weakest part of a steam sterilizer is the
    c. *door.* *(14 / 305)*

32. Because shelf life is event related, stock rotation is no longer necessary.
    b. *False* *(16 / 352)*

33. Aluminum foil is an approved packaging material for use in ethylene oxide sterilizers.
    b. *False* *(15 / 327)*

34. Stainless steel jaw needle holders last longer than tungsten carbide jaw needle holders.
    b. *False* *(10 / 186)*

35. Endoscopes are often processed in a mechanical unit called
    d. *an automatic endoscope reprocessor.* *(11 / 227)*

36. Which of the following is NOT an acceptable sterilization packaging material?
    c. *Canvas* *(12 / 260)*

37. Phenolics are classified as
    a. *intermediate- to low-level disinfectants.* *(9 / 165)*

38. Cleaning is defined as the removal of all visible and non-visible soil.
    a. *True* *(8 / 130)*

39. Standards and regulations help set
    a. *minimal levels of quality and safety.* *(5 / 86)*

40. When it is necessary to transport soiled items between facilities using a truck or van, facilities must consult U.S. Department of Transportation, as well as state and local laws for transporting biohazardous items.
    a. *True* *(7 / 127)*

41. Which of the following is NOT a requirement of the Occupational Safety and Health Administration Bloodborne Pathogen Standard?
    c. *Keep biohazard areas locked* *(6 / 111)*

42. Due to the difficulty of cleaning items contaminated with prions
      d. *all of the above.*   *(4 / 82)*

43. Arthroscopy means
      a. *visual exam of a joint.*   *(2 / 28)*

44. The hip joint is an example of a
      b. *ball and socket joint.*   *(3 / 44)*

45. All items sterilized or high-level disinfected at the point of use must be carefully monitored and logged.
      a. *True*   *(13 / 297)*

46. When loading a steam sterilizer
      d. *do all of the above.*   *(14 / 315)*

47. One of the goals of stock arrangement is to provide minimal product handling while allowing first in, first out rotation.
      a. *True*   *(16 / 352)*

48. What exposure monitoring is required for all personnel using a hydrogen peroxide sterilizer?
      a. *No monitoring is required*   *(15 / 330-34)*

49. To properly test the sharpness of scissors four inches or less use
      a. *yellow test material.*   *(10 / 196)*

50. Loaner instrumentation can cause receiving challenges.
      a. *True*   *(11 / 239)*

51. When placing instruments in a peel pack, the tips should always face the paper side of the pack.
      b. *False*   *(12 / 268)*

52. When mixing several low- to intermediate-level disinfectants together, it is important to remember
      d. *chemicals should not be mixed.*   *(9 / 172)*

53. Powered surgical instruments should be cleaned using a mechanical cleaning process.
      b. *False*   *(8 / 156)*

54. Following Occupational Safety and Health Administration regulations for wearing personal protective equipment in the Central Service decontamination area is optional.
      b. *False*   *(5 / 93)*

55. It is acceptable to transport soiled and clean items at the same time in the same cart if they are placed on separate shelves.
      b. *False*   *(7 / 125)*

56. What color should biohazard labels/signs be?
      a. *Red/orange*   *(6 / 111)*

57. Microorganisms reproduce by a process called
      b. *binary fission.*   *(4 / 76)*

58. Not understanding medical terminology may compromise patient care.
    a.   True   *(2 / 22)*

59. This the first step in the sterilization process.
    d.   Cleaning   *(1 / 10)*

60. This surgical procedure is the removal of the gall bladder.
    a.   Cholecystectomy   *(3 / 62)*

61. When transporting items that have been immediate use steam sterilized, it is required that
    d.   they be transported in such a manner that reduces the potential for
        contamination.   *(13 / 296)*

62. Using the wrong container filter or poor filter placement can be a cause of a wet pack.
    a.   True   *(14 / 318)*

63. Heavy items should be placed
    c.   on the middle shelves.   *(16 / 350)*

64. Lumens should be moist, using hydrogen peroxide as an agent, when sterilized.
    b.   False   *(15 / 331)*

65. Outside shipping containers
    a.   should be removed prior to placing the items in storage.   *(16 / 348)*

66. Microgrind or supercut scissors are usually identified with a black handle.
    a.   True   *(10 / 191)*

67. The purpose of the insulation covering laparoscopy instruments is to
    c.   protect the patient from electrical current.   *(11 / 217)*

68. Airflow in the prep and pack area should be
    b.   positive.   *(12 / 244)*

69. The process by which all forms of microorganisms are completely destroyed is called
    c.   sterilization.   *(9 / 163)*

70. What is the most common pH for detergents used for most cleaning processes?
    c.   neutral pH.   *(8 / 147)*

71. Surgical instruments are carefully inspected for cleanliness and function in
    the _____area of the Central Service department.
    d.   preparation and packaging   *(1 / 11)*

72. This surgical procedure consists of removing an ear bone that has thickened and no longer transmits sound waves and replacing it with an artificial implant to improve hearing.
    b.   Stapedectomy   *(3 / 53)*

73. Multiple drug resistant organisms are a declining threat to patients in healthcare facilities.
    b.   False   *(4 / 76)*

74. The root element *gastro* refers to the
    d.   stomach.   *(2 / 30)*

75. Point-of-use preparation
    b. begins the cleaning process.   (7 / 122)

76. The only way to interrupt the transmission of a causative agent is to
    c. eliminate it.   (6 / 115)

77. Which of the following statements about Immediate Use Steam Sterilization is true?
    d. It should be used only when there is not time to process items using the
        wrapped method.   (13 / 293)

78. The guidelines for sterile storages are the same for both items sterilized in house
    and for items purchased sterile.
    a. True   (16 / 349)

79. Information about a device's compatibility with a specific sterilization process
    should be obtained from the device's manufacturer.
    a. True   (15 / 324)

80. The higher the bioburden on an object
    a. the more difficult it will be to sterilize.   (14 / 302)

81. Sterile storage areas should
    b. have positive airflow and at least four air exchanges per hour. (16 / 344)

82. The part of a hemostat that locks and holds it in position is called the box lock.
    b. False   (10 / 183)

83. The purpose of a decontamination battery is to protect powered surgical
    instruments from fluid invasion.
    a. True   (11 / 210)

84. Temperature in the preparation and packaging area should be
    c. between 68 and 73 degrees Fahrenheit.   (12 / 244)

85. In an automated washer the key source of disinfection is
    b. water temperature.   (9 / 173)

86. Written cleaning instructions for surgical instruments should be provided by
    b. the device manufacturer.   (8 / 149)

87. In the future, which of the following will more frequently become a
    requirement for working in a Central Service department?
    c. Formal education   (1 / 19)

88. More than 55% of blood is made up of this yellowish liquid.
    d. Plasma   (3 / 63)

89. Bacteria that require free oxygen are called
    c. aerobic.   (4 / 75)

90. The suffix -ectomy means
    a. surgical removal.   (2 / 28)

91. To prevent coagulation of proteins, instruments should be pre-rinsed using
    a. cool water.   (8 / 142)

92. Regulations and standards provide information to help ensure
    a. *quality and safety.* *(5 / 86)*

93. When assembling instrument trays
    a. *heavier instruments should be placed on the bottom of the tray.* *(12 / 255)*

94. Devices categorized as semi-critical items, must be at least _____ prior to use.
    a. *high-level disinfected* *(9 / 162)*

95. The human resources tool that identifies major tasks performed by persons in specific positions is called a
    d. *job description.* *(1 / 18)*

96. This gland stimulates body growth.
    d. *Pituitary gland* *(3/ 54)*

97. The steam sterilization process can be affected by the design of the medical device being sterilized.
    a. *True* *(14 / 302)*

98. Ethylene oxide, hydrogen peroxide and ozone sterilization process must all be monitored using chemical, physical and biological monitors.
    a. *True* *(15 / 323)*

99. Kerrison/laminectomy rongeurs should be tested using
    d. *an index card.* *(10 / 196)*

100. Flexible endoscopes that fail a leak test may continue to be used until the break/hole impacts the scope's function.
    b. *False* *(11 / 223)*

Progress Test Five   *chapter/page*

1. Temperature and humidity levels need to be monitored and recorded
    c. *at least daily.* *(17 / 359)*

2. Survey readiness is the responsibility of
    a. *every Central Service technician.* *(18 / 387)*

3. Product expiration dates are located on this part of each package.
    d. *There is no standard place to look for an expiration date* *(19 / 397)*

4. If an equipment malfunction causes harm to patients, it should be
    d. *returned immediately to the Biomedical department.* *(20 / 411)*

5. One type of formal monitoring is watching the department's temperature and humidity levels.
    a. *True* *(17 / 359)*

6. Occupational Safety and Health Administration is responsible for
    a. *ethylene oxide guidelines, worker safety, and the bloodborne pathogen standard.* *(5 / 92-93)*

7. The ears are made up of three parts
    a. *inner, exterior and middle.* *(3 / 51)*

8. The most common reason steam sterilization failure is
   a. *lack of steam contact with the instrument.* *(14 / 311)*

9. When using glutaraldehyde technicians should always wear latex gloves for protection.
   b. *False* *(9 / 168)*

10. Using latex tubing to protect delicate instrumentation is the process of choice for items to be steam sterilized.
    b. *False* *(12 / 253)*

11. The purpose of using a decontamination battery or hose when cleaning powered surgical instruments is
    a. *to keep fluid from entering the unit.* *(11 / 208 & 210)*

12. Healthcare-associated infections are
    d. *infections which occur in the course of being treated in a healthcare facility.* *(1 / 28)*

13. Items that have been used in patient care should be considered contaminated.
    a. *True* *(7 / 126)*

14. The term *excise* means
    c. *to cut out.* *(2 / 18)*

15. Water must be degassed each time the ultrasonic cleaner's tank is changed because
    a. *excess bubbles from filling reduce the energy of the cavitation process.* *(8 / 140)*

16. Wrapped trays should not be stacked because
    b. *the trays will be damaged.* *(16 / 347)*

17. Woven reusable fabrics are the packaging products of choice for ozone sterilization.
    b. *False* *(15 / 336)*

18. Instrument lubrication should be performed
    b. *following the manufacturer's Instructions for Use.* *(10 / 199)*

19. Documentation is not required for items that are immediate use steam sterilized.
    b. *False* *(13 / 297)*

20. Microbes
    d. *are all of the above* *(4 / 71)*

21. Each year, approximately _____ patients develop a healthcare-associated infection.
    c. *700,000* *(6 / 102)*

22. Monitoring records must be
    d. *all the above.* *(17 / 358)*

23. Always wearing personal protective equipment in the decontamination area is a quality process.
    a. *True* *(18 / 387)*

24. Case cart systems
    a. *reduce the amount of inventory needed in user departments.* *(19 / 401)*

25. Which of the following requires preventive maintenance standards be established for medical equipment?
    b. The Joint Commission   (20 / 410)

26. In order to reprocess single-use devices, a hospital must be able to prove the device will act the same as it did when it was first manufactured.
    a. True   (5 / 90)

27. The iris is
    b. the colored portion of the eye.   (3 / 50)

28. Three of the main phases of a terminal steam sterilizer cycle are
    d. conditioning, exposure and exhaust.   (14 / 308)

29. The use of heat to kill all microorganisms, except spores, is called
    b. thermal disinfection.   (9 / 173)

30. Clean multi-part instruments that have been assembled to test for functionality should
    c. be disassembled and sterilized following manufacturer's
        Instructions for Use.   (12 / 249)

31. The endoscope that would be dispensed for a procedure that required visualization of the lower part of the large intestine would be a
    b. sigmoidoscope.   (11 / 221)

32. Central Service technicians must wear special attire referred to as _____ to minimize their exposure to bloodborne pathogens and other contaminants.
    a. PPE   (1 / 11)

33. To help prevent the growth of biofilm, soil on used instruments should be allowed to dry.
    b. False   (7 / 126)

34. The suffix *plasty*
    c. is a suffix meaning surgical restoration.   (2 / 29)

35. Using untreated water
    a. increases the likelihood of mineral scale deposits.   (8 / 135)

36. Sterile trays should
    d. all the above.   (16 / 347)

37. Ethylene oxide is a toxic gas.
    a. True   (15 / 325)

38. Scissors with tungsten carbide cutting edges are usually identified by
    c. gold handles.   (10 / 190)

39. The sterilization method of choice for single-use items is immediate use steam sterilization.
    b. False   (13 / 295)

40. The basic unit of a living organism
    a. cells.   (4 / 71)

41. Know what is dirty, know what is clean, know what is sterile; keeping the three conditions separate, and remedying contamination immediately are
    a. *the principles of asepsis.*   *(6 / 104)*

42. Documentation of immediate use steam sterilization cycles should include
    a. *patient identification and reason for the immediate use steam sterilization cycle.*   *(17 / 369)*

43. A true Central Service quality program utilizes
    a. *all Central Service personnel and a cross section of its customers.*   *(18 / 376)*

44. Requisition systems are primarily used in large facilities.
    b. *False*   *(19 / 400)*

45. When Central Service supports affiliated clinics
    c. *planning and communication are is critical.*   *(20 / 415)*

46. Class III medical devices are identified as high risk.
    a. *True*   *(5 / 89)*

47. An organ that filters the blood to remove amino acids and some harmful toxins
    c. *liver.*   *(3 / 58)*

48. Immediate use steam sterilization is the process to sterilize trays for future use.
    b. *False*   *(14 / 308)*

49. Which of the following are classified as high-level disinfectants?
    b. *Glutaraldehyde and ortho-phthalaldehydes*   *(9 / 170)*

50. The U.S. Food and Drug Administration classifies sterilization packaging as a
    b. *Class II medical device.*   *(12 / 259)*

51. Loaner instruments should
    c. *be decontaminated before use.*   *(11 / 240)*

52. Maintaining professional conduct standards and adapting to changing situations are examples of
    d. *employability skills.*   *(1 / 16)*

53. Users are responsible to notify Central Service if they discover instruments or equipment that are in need of repair.
    a. *True*   *(7 / 124)*

54. The term *ostomy*
    b. *is a suffix.*   *(2 / 28)*

55. Instrument lubrication is performed
    c. *after cleaning.*   *(8 / 149)*

56. The bottom shelf of any sterile storage system should be
    a. *solid and eight to 10 inches from the floor.*   *(16 / 346)*

57. Cellulose-containing packaging materials are not compatible with hydrogen peroxide sterilization.
    a. *True*   *(15 / 331 & 334)*

58. The purpose of a suction stylet is to
    a. *unclog the suction during surgery.*   *(10 / 191)*

59. It is recommended to use immediate use steam sterilization to sterilize instruments contaminated with Creutzfeldt-Jakob disease after the procedure has been completed.
    b. *False*   *(13 / 295)*

60. Bacteria that cause disease are called
    c. *pathogens.*   *(4 / 71)*

61. Asepsis is defined as
    d. *the absence of microorganisms that cause disease.*   *(6 / 104)*

62. External indicators can prove an item is sterile when the sterilization cycle is complete.
    b. *False*   *(17 / 362)*

63. The degree or grade of excellence of a product or service is called
    d. *quality.*   *(18 / 374)*

64. Capital equipment items are items
    a. *with a high cost.*   *(19 / 393)*

65. Which of the following statements is correct?
    c. *Tracking patient care equipment can prevent equipment shortages*   *(20 / 413)*

66. Medical device reporting is regulated by the
    d. *U.S. Food and Drug Administration.*   *(5 / 88)*

67. This surgical procedure removes tissue or displaced bone from the wrist area to release pressure on the median nerve.
    a. *Carpal tunnel repair*   *(3 / 52)*

68. Steam flush pressure pulse sterilizers are a type of gravity sterilizers.
    b. *False*   *(14 / 307)*

69. Thermal disinfection is accomplished using
    d. *heat.*   *(9 / 173)*

70. When placing instruments in a peel pack, the tips should always face the paper side of the pack.
    b. *False*   *(12 / 268)*

71. Information regarding cleaning processes for endoscopes should be provided by
    c. *the instrument manufacturer.*   *(11 / 222)*

72. Which of the following is an advantage of minimally invasive surgery?
    b. *Shorter recovery times*   *(1 / 8)*

73. When moving transport carts throughout the healthcare facility, Central Service technicians must always yield right of way to patients and visitors.
    a. *True*   *(7 / 126)*

74. The last word element in a medical term is the
    c. *suffix.*   *(2 / 24)*

75. Instruments should be cleaned using a
    b. *to and fro motion.* *(8 / 153)*

76. Trays that overhang the shelving
    a. *can become contaminated.* *(16 / 344)*

77. An extended aeration cycle is required for items sterilized in ozone sterilization processes.
    b. *False* *(15 / 335)*

78. Instrument marking tape should be wrapped approximately _____ around the instrument.
    a. *1.5 times* *(10 / 198)*

79. Items to be disinfected or sterilized at point of use must be
    a. *properly cleaned per manufacturer's Instructions for Use.* *(13 / 292 & 298)*

80. _____ is an example of a fungus.
    c. *Athlete's foot* *(4 / 80)*

81. Hand hygiene means hands are kept germ free at work.
    b. *False* *(6 / 105)*

82. A biological indicator is called positive when
    c. *when there is growth in the ampule after incubation.* *(17 / 364)*

83. Quality planning includes studying other facilities.
    a. *True* *(18 / 377)*

84. The inventory system that stocks supplies by established stock levels is called
    a. *a periodic automated replenishment system.* *(19 / 399)*

85. All patient care equipment that was dispensed for use must be considered
    _____, and handled as such, regardless of its appearance.
    c. *contaminated* *(20 / 411)*

86. Agency which imposes very strict labeling requirements on manufacturers of chemicals used by Central Service departments.
    c. *Environmental Protection Agency* *(5 / 92)*

87. The largest part of the human brain is the
    c. *cerebrum.* *(3 / 49)*

88. The coolest place in a steam sterilizer is
    b. *the thermostatic valve.* *(14 / 306)*

89. How long must alcohol remain in wet contact with an item to achieve a reasonable level of disinfection?
    c. *Five to 10 minutes* *(9/ 165)*

90. Temperatures in a sterile storage area should be 55 to 60 degrees Fahrenheit.
    b. *False* *(16 / 344)*

91. All flexible endoscopes have internal channels.
    b. *False* *(11 / 221)*

92. While items may be dispensed to all areas of a facility, the major focus of the sterile storage personnel is
    d. the Operating Room.   (1 / 13)

93. The following symbolizes

    d. product manufacture date.   (19 / 396)

94. Everyone who may transport contaminated items must be trained in safe handling procedures.
    a. True   (7 / 125)

95. The purpose of a combining vowel is to
    c. ease pronunciation of a word.   (2 / 24)

96. Instruments received from surgery and tagged for repair do not need to be cleaned until they come back from repair.
    b. False   (8 / 154)

97. Customer surveys are ineffective tools in establishing Central Service quality processes.
    b. False   (18 / 375)

98. Which of the following systems provides supplies and instruments for individual surgical procedures?
    c. Case cart   (19 / 401)

99. The shelving system of choice for the sterile storage area is
    a. closed.   (16 / 345)

100. Aluminum foil is an approved packaging material for use in ethylene oxide sterilizers.
    b. False   (15 / 327)

101. After applying instrument identification tape, instruments should be autoclaved to help the tape bond to the instrument.
    a. True   (10 / 198)

102. Both Association of perioperative Registered Nurses and The Joint Commission recommend that
    a. the use of immediate use steam sterilization be minimized or decreased.   (13 / 293-94)

103. The part of a cell that controls cell function is the
    b. nucleus.   (4 / 71)

104. When putting on personal protective equipment it is important to put the mask on first.
    b. False   (6 / 109)

105. Washer disinfector screens should be cleaned at least
    a. daily.   (8 / 143)

106. The Hospital Consumer Assessment of Healthcare Providers and Systems
    b. *is designed to evaluate hospital stays from a patient's perception.*   *(18 / 386)*

107. This program is designed to reduce harm to the environment
    c. *sustainability.*   *(19 / 404)*

108. The decision to use reusable or disposable instruments in procedure trays is determined by
    d. *amount of items to be used and delivery schedules.*   *(20 / 415)*

109. Cartilage is replaced by bone through a process called
    a. *ossification.*   *(3 / 44)*

110. The steam sterilization process can be affected by the types of soil present on the devices to be sterilized.
    a. *True*   *(14 / 302)*

111. These chemicals are used on animate (living tissue) to slow the growth of microorganisms
    d. *antiseptics.*   *(9 / 165)*

112. Cellulose materials cannot be processed within a hydrogen peroxide sterilizer.
    a. *True*   *(12 / 266)*

113. Temperature and humidity levels in the sterile storage area should be checked and recorded at least weekly.
    b. *False*   *(16 / 344)*

114. Ethylene oxide, hydrogen peroxide and ozone sterilization can all use the same packaging materials.
    b. *False*   *(15 / 327, 331, 334)*

115. Preference cards are used with a requisition inventory system.
    b. *False*   *(19 / 401)*

116. Preventive maintenance
    b. *is designed to identify potential problems before they occur.*   *(20 / 414)*

117. Increased education helps technicians provide higher quality services.
    a. *True*   *(18 / 375)*

118. Which of the following common items of patient care equipment limits the development of deep vein thrombosis and peripheral edema in immobile patients?
    c. *Sequential compression unit*   *(20 / 409)*

119. Central Service technicians need to understand the anatomy of a steam sterilizer
    b. *to understand how the sterilizer operates.*   *(14 / 303)*

120. The spore is the control unit of a cell.
    b. *False*   *(4 / 71)*

121. The main theory of standard precautions is
    d. *to treat all human blood and body fluids as infectious.*   *(6 / 103)*

122. The International Standards Organization uses routine and unannounced inspections to monitor standards in healthcare facilities.
    b. *False*   *(18 / 386)*

123. The U.S. Food and Drug Administration Class II chemical indicator run daily in dynamic air removal sterilizers is called
    d. *Bowie-Dick test.* *(17 / 368)*

124. Equipment should be inspected for obvious hazards such as cracked or frayed electrical cords
    d. *whenever the equipment is inspected in Central Service.* *(20 / 410)*

125. Documentation log sheets should be maintained when using a high-level disinfectant.
    a. *True* *(9 / 176)*

126. Many words may contain more than one root element.
    a. *True* *(2 / 24)*

127. Horizontal work surfaces in the decontamination area should be cleaned and disinfected once per day.
    b. *False* *(8 / 133)*

128. Accessories for electric powered equipment include
    b. *foot switches.* *(11 / 206)*

129. The use of analytical skills to solve problems and make decisions is a component of which of the following knowledge and skills dimensions?
    c. *Employability skills* *(1 / 16)*

130. One of the goals of point-of-use preparation and transport is to
    c. *prevent cross contamination.* *(7 / 120)*

131. Automated supply replenishment systems are
    d. *computerized.* *(19 / 399)*

132. Most powered surgical instruments are immiscible.
    b. *False* *(11 / 206, 208, 209)*

133. The sterile storage process starts
    c. *when the sterilizer door is opened.* *(16 / 342)*

134. The place where the two parts of an instrument meet and pivot is called the box lock.
    a. *True* *(10 / 183)*

135. When sterilizing items at point of use an abbreviated sterilization cycle may be used due to the urgent need for the instruments.
    b. *False* *(13 / 295)*

136. Technicians in the _____ department perform safety inspections and functional tests on equipment.
    c. *Biomedical Engineering* *(20 / 410)*

137. The inventory system that uses two identical carts to facilitate supply replenishment is called the
    b. *exchange cart system.* *(19 / 400)*

138. All department staff members must be fully engaged to make a quality program successful.
    a. *True* *(18 / 378)*

139. Chemical indicators can show a fail result because of
    d. all the above.   *(17 / 363)*

140. Pyrogens
    a. are fever-producing substances.   *(8 / 135)*

Progress Test Six   <u>*chapter/page*</u>

1. Information technology is often the cornerstone of initiatives to transform healthcare.
    a. True   *(21 / 419)*

2. Disposable items increase combustible load in a healthcare facility.
    a. True   *(22 / 438)*

3. Enabling people to use information gained to interact with others is known as
    a. human relations.   *(23 / 452)*

4. At this time, tracking systems are unable to track worker productivity information.
    b. False   *(21 / 426)*

5. A step in communication that occurs when a listener asks a question is called
    b. feedback.   *(23 / 455)*

6. Improving your professional development skills is an important part of
    d. career advancement.   *(24 / 469)*

7. The U.S. Food and Drug Administration Class II chemical indicator run daily in dynamic air removal sterilizers is called a
    d. Bowie-Dick test.   *(17 / 368)*

8. Always wearing personal protective equipment in the decontamination area is a quality process.
    a. True   *(18 / 387)*

9. Product expiration dates are located on this part of each package.
    d. There is no standard place to look for an expiration date   *(19 / 397)*

10. When patient equipment enters a healthcare facility, it must be safety checked by a _____before it is cleared for patient use.
    a. Biomedical technician   *(20 / 410)*

11. These are used to breakdown fatty tissue on instruments
    b. lipase enzymes.   *(8 / 146)*

12. Anaerobic bacteria require free oxygen to live.
    b. False   *(4 / 72)*

13. The absence of microorganisms that cause disease is called
    c. asepsis.   *(6 / 104)*

14. Immediate use steam sterilization was developed to process items when the facility does not have enough instruments to perform the surgery.
    b. False   *(13 / 294)*

15. When an instrument has a shiny surface it is said to have a _____ finish.
    d. mirror   *(10 / 183)*

16. Lumens should be moist when sterilized using hydrogen peroxide as a sterilizing agent.
    b. *False*   *(15 / 331)*

17. Most Central Service departments employ some sort of automated Information management system.
    a. *True*   *(21 / 418)*

18. Ethylene oxide gas canisters should be stored
    a. *in a containment locker.*   *(22 / 443)*

19. Knowing what is expected and consistently meeting those expectations are part of
    d. *professional behavior.*   *(23 / 454)*

20. Improving employability skills requires
    c. *identifying requirements for your goal.*   *(24 / 468)*

21. Sterile packages should be stored no lower than eight to 10 inches from the floor.
    a. *True*   *(16 / 346)*

22. Combining vowels are used to
    a. *help with the pronunciation of the word.*   *(2 / 24)*

23. If soiled instruments are to be transported to an offsite facility for processing
    c. *they should be transported following the U.S. or state Department of Transportation guidelines.*   *(7 / 127)*

24. The decontamination area of the Central Service department is where instruments are carefully checked for cleanliness and function.
    b. *False*   *(1 / 10)*

25. Arthroscopy instruments are used during
    c. *joint surgery.*   *(11 / 219)*

26. Some plastics including formulations of spun-bonded polyolefin are intended for use in these sterilization processes
    b. *ozone and hydrogen peroxide.*   *(12 / 266)*

27. The amount of time an item must remain wet with a disinfectant to achieve disinfection is called.
    b. *Wet contact time*   *(9 / 173)*

28. The drain screen in a steam sterilizer must be cleaned
    c. *at least daily.*   *(14 / 305)*

29. This surgical procedure removes the uterus.
    b. *Hysterectomy*   *(3 / 56)*

30. Recommendations regarding sterilization practices are provided by the Association for the Advancement of Medical Instrumentation.
    a. *True*   *(5 / 95)*

31. Which of the following is NOT a result of computer integration?
    c. *Automatically provides critical update to industry standards*   *(21 / 419)*

32. A plane crash is an example of an external disaster.
    a. *True*   *(22 / 447)*

33. Effective communication skills will resolve all communication problems.
    b. *False*   *(23 / 453)*

34. Professional development is a commitment to continuous learning.
    a. True   *(24 / 468)*

35. In addition to providing financial and operational management, information technology systems are used to help ensure patient safety.
    a. True   *(21 / 419)*

36. Which of the following is true about a valuing diversity effort?
    d. *None of the above statements is correct*   *(23 / 463)*

37. Safety relates to freedom from damage, risk or injury.
    a. True   *(22 / 430)*

39. Personal development is mandatory while professional development is only needed for career advancement.
    b. *False*   *(24 / 469)*

39. Employee training should occur
    d. *for both new employees and employees who moves to a new position.*   *(17 / 371)*

40. If everyone develops a quality-driven focus, written policies and procedures are not necessary in the Central Service department.
    b. *False*   *(18 / 386)*

41. The movement of supplies throughout the healthcare facility is called
    a. *distribution.*   *(19 / 398)*

42. All patient care equipment that was dispensed for use must be considered _____, and handled as such, regardless of its appearance.
    c. *contaminated*   *(20 / 411)*

43. What is the preferred pH for detergents used for most cleaning processes?
    c. *Neutral pH*   *(8 / 147)*

44. All microorganisms are harmful to humans.
    b. *False*   *(4 / 71)*

45. Inanimate objects that can transmit bacteria are called
    b. *fomites.*   *(6 / 113)*

46. All items sterilized or high-level disinfected at point of use must be carefully monitored and logged.
    a. True   *(13 / 297-98)*

47. Instrument marking tape should be wrapped approximately _____ around the instrument.
    a. *1.5 times*   *(10 / 198)*

48. Hydrogen peroxide kills microorganisms by a process called oxidation.
    a. True   *(15 / 323)*

49. Event related shelf life means items are safe until opened for use.
    b. *False*   *(16 / 349)*

50. The term *ectomy* means
    b. *surgical removal.*   *(2 / 28)*

51. The proper handling of instrumentation is the responsibility of
    d. *everyone who comes in contact with the instrumentation.* *(7 / 122)*

52. A pick list contains information that
    d. *identifies the supplies and instruments needed for a specific doctor
       and procedure.* *(1 / 13-14)*

53. After use, loaner instrumentation must be decontaminated before it is shipped
    back to the vendor.
    a. *True* *(11 / 241)*

54. Cellulose materials cannot be processed within a hydrogen peroxide sterilizer.
    a. *True* *(12 /266)*

55. Which of the following would be the best choice for high-level disinfection of instruments?
    d. *Ortho-phthalaldehydes* *(9 / 169)*

56. The steam sterilization process can be affected by the design of the medical device
    being sterilized.
    a. *True* *(14 / 302)*

57. Organs are two or more cells that are similar.
    b. *False* *(3 / 43)*

58. Which organization writes standards relating to the processing of flexible endoscopes?
    a. *The Society of Gastroenterology Nurses and Associates* *(5 / 98)*

59. Which of these traffic control/dress code requirements applies to the clean
    assembly area of Central Service?
    c. *Semi restricted* *(6 / 110)*

60. Computerized tracking systems are fast, but manual tracking systems are more
    effective for tracking.
    b. *False* *(21 / 424)*

61. Which of the following information is NOT included on a safety data sheet?
    c. *Required inventory levels* *(22 / 436)*

62. Customer complaints are best handled through which of the following approaches?
    c. *Being cheerful and courteous* *(23 / 464)*

63. Networking inside your profession can help you increase your knowledge toward
    advancement while networking outside your profession does not.
    b. *False* *(24 / 471)*

64. Which of the following is NOT a feature of an instrument tracking system?
    d. *Product updates and recall information* *(21 / 426)*

65. This process allows a person to understand someone else's needs.
    a. *Communication* *(23/ 452)*

66. Safety data sheets are provided by
    d. *the product manufacturer.* *(22 / 436)*

67. One important step in preparing for an interview is
    c. *anticipating possible interview questions.* *(24 / 473)*

68. Sterilizer load records should contain
    a. items and quantity sterilized.   *(17 / 366)*

69. The quality method failure mode and effects analysis is a
    d. quality method to prevent problems before they occur.   *(18 / 379)*

70. A disadvantage of an exchange cart system is
    d. they require duplicate inventory.   *(19 / 400)*

71. Patient care equipment should be stored in a _____ condition.
    a. "ready to dispense"   *(20 / 412)*

72. Cleaning brushes
    a. should be cleaned and sterilized at least daily.   *(8 / 137)*

73. Microbiology is the study of
    b. microorganisms.   *(4 / 70)*

74. The basics of aseptic technique
    b. are activities that prevent infection.   *(6/ 104)*

75. To sterilize items using immediate use steam sterilization, the item's manufacturer instructions must state the item can be sterilized using an immediate use steam sterilization cycle.
    a. True   *(13 / 294)*

76. Laser finished instruments are coated with a durable protective finish that cannot be chipped or scratched.
    b. False   *(10 / 200)*

77. Information about a device's compatibility with a specific sterilization process should be obtained from the device's manufacturer.
    a. True   *(15 / 324)*

78. Temperatures in the sterile storage area should be 64 to 78° Fahrenheit.
    b. False   *(16 / 344)*

79. The suffix *tome* means
    d. cutting instrument.   *(2 / 29)*

80. It is acceptable to transport soiled and clean items at the same time in the same cart if they are placed on separate shelves.
    b. False   *(7 / 125)*

81. Soiled instruments and other items are received in the _____ area of the Central Service department.
    c. decontamination   *(1 / 10)*

82. Which of the following should be used to thoroughly rinse (remove) all traces of disinfectant from an endoscope's channels?
    c. Treated water   *(11 / 225)*

83. When placing instruments that open in an instrument tray, you should
    d. unlock the handles and open the instruments.   *(12/ 253)*

84. Items that are introduced directly into the bloodstream or other normally sterile areas of the body are classified as
    a. critical items.   *(9 / 162)*

85. Gravity steam sterilizers use a pump or water injector to remove air from the chamber.
    b.   *False*   *(14 / 307)*

86. The procedure to remove the stomach is
    b.   *gastrectomy.*   *(3 / 61)*

87. Failure to receive accreditation from The Joint Commission can result in the loss of Medicare and Medicaid payments.
    a.   *True*   *(5 / 97)*

88. Which of the following tracking methods provides real-time information?
    a.   *Radio frequency identification tags*   *(21 / 423)*

89. Healthcare facilities using ethylene oxide should have a dedicated ventilation system to remove residual ethylene oxide during the exhaust cycle.
    a.   *True*   *(22 / 443)*

90. Which of the following is an example of communication?
    d.   *All of the above*   *(23 / 452)*

91. Professional development skill building activities include
    d.   *all the above.*   *(24 / 472)*

93. A group of employees from different departments within the healthcare facility that work together to solve operating problems is called a
    c.   *cross-functional team.*   *(23 / 462)*

93. Which of the following is NOT a component of risk management?
    c.   *Staff management*   *(22 / 430)*

94. Planning and reviewing your goals will help identify activities to help you meet those goals.
    a.   *True*   *(24 / 470)*

95. Documentation of immediate use steam sterilization cycles should include
    a.   *patient identification and reason for the immediate use steam sterilization cycle.*   *(17 / 369)*

96. Quality requires the efforts and participation of everyone in the healthcare facility.
    a.   *True*   *(18 / 375)*

97. Supplies such as disposable wraps are called
    a.   *consumable.*   *(19 / 393)*

98. Preventive maintenance
    b.   *is designed to identify potential problems before they occur.*   *(20 / 414)*

99. Detergents used in mechanical cleaners should be
    d.   *low foaming.*   *(8 / 148)*

100. When cleaning prion contaminated instruments no special cleaning procedures are required only following standard cleaning protocols and the manufacturer's Instructions for Use.
    b.   *False*   *(4 / 82)*

101. Hand hygiene is considered the single most important factor in reducing infections.
    a.   *True*   *(6 / 105)*

102. Immediate use steam sterilization documentation should include
    d.   *all the above.*   *(13 / 297)*

103. An osteotome is
   a.   used to cut or shave bone.   (10 / 182)

104. Woven reusable fabrics are the packaging products of choice for ozone sterilization.
   b.   False   (15 / 336)

105. Sterile items should be stored at least _____ inches below sprinkler heads.
   b.   18   (16 / 350)

106. Which of the following means *beside* or *near*?
   a.   Para   (2 / 33)

107. Decontamination of instruments and equipment starts
   c.   at the point of use.   (7 / 121)

108. All Central Service departments perform the same basic services.
   b.   False   (1 / 9)

109. Leak testing should be performed on each flexible endoscope annually.
   b.   False   (11 / 223)

110. When placing instruments in a peel pack, the tips should always face the paper side of the pack.
   b.   False   (12 / 268)

111. Devices listed as critical items, must be _____ prior to use.
   d.   sterilized   (9 / 162)

112. When combining loads, hard goods should be placed on the top shelves to allow for more efficient removal of the condensate.
   b.   False   (14 / 315)

113. Items that are wrapped moist can be a cause of wet packs.
   a.   True   (14 / 318)

114. A herniorrhaphy surgical procedure is
   b.   repair of a muscle layer that is allowing all or part of an organ to project through an opening.   (3 / 48)

115. Voluntary standards
   b.   provide guidelines for better patient care.   (5 / 86)

116. Tracking individual instruments is important to help ensure specific instruments are kept with a specific set.
   a.   True   (21 / 425)

117. Personal headsets should not be used in the Central Service department because they
   b.   reduce the ability to hear telephones, alarms and coworkers.   (23 / 459)

118. Which of the following is NOT required for sharps safety?
   c.   Wash all disposable sharps before discarding them   (22 / 434)

119. On the job relationships do not change when one team member has been promoted.
   b.   False   (24 / 474)

120. Hospitals can effectively validate sterilization processes.
   c.   False   (17 / 367)